BROKEN PROMISES

BROKEN PROMISES

How the AIDS Establishment Has Betrayed the Developing World

EDWARD C. GREEN

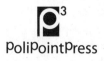

PoliPointPress

Broken Promises: How the AIDS Establishment Has
Betrayed the Developing World

Copyright © 2011 by Edward C. Green

15   14   13   12   11   1   2   3   4   5

Production management: BookMatters
Book design: BookMatters
Cover design: Naylor Design, Inc.

Library of Congress Cataloging-in-Publication Data
Green, Edward C. (Edward Crocker), 1944–
  Broken promises : how the AIDS establishment has
betrayed the developing world / Edward C. Green.
    p. ; cm.
  Includes bibliographical references and index.
  ISBN 978-1-936227-00-6 (alk. paper)
    1. AIDS (Disease)—Africa—Prevention. I. Title.
  [DNLM: 1. Developing Countries—Africa.
  2. HIV Infections—prevention & control—Africa.
  3. HIV Infections—epidemiology—Africa.
  4. Health Knowledge, Attitudes, Practice—Africa.
  5. International Cooperation—Africa. WC 503.6]
  RA643.86.A35G74   2011
  362.19'97920096—dc22   2010044897

Published by:
PoliPointPress, LLC
80 Liberty Ship Way, Suite 22
Sausalito, CA 94965
(415) 339-4100
www.p3books.com

Distributed by Ingram Publisher Services

Printed in the USA

Unanswered questions are far less dangerous than unquestioned answers.

—UNKNOWN

Contents

Prologue   ix

Part I **THE ROAD TO FIDELITY**

  1 Gangs, Maroons, and the Egg Taboo   3
  2 The Visitation   15

Part II **UGANDA**

  3 The Twenty-five-cent Solution   29
  4 The Crossroads and the Cul-de-sac   45
  5 Infidelity   65

Part III **CALAMITY'S CRADLE**

  6 Putting the Bedroom before the Sickroom   77
  7 Ins and Outs of the Castle   107

Part IV **SHIFTING THE RIVERBED**

  8 Jihad   133
  9 Breakthrough   145
  10 Policy by Applause   163

11 Cracking the Error Edifice   185
12 Chasing the Wild Programs   201
13 A Bridge to Somewhere?   211

    Epilogue   225
    Abbreviations and Acronyms   233
    Notes   235
    Index   253
    About the Author   268

Prologue

It is the response to error that counts.

NIKKI GIOVANNI
"Of Liberation"

In the spring of 2009, Pope Benedict XVI was flying to Africa on Shepherd One. You may have ridden on it yourself, because the Vatican simply borrows whatever airliner Alitalia has available when the Pope goes abroad. His small staff, a security detail, and seventy-odd journalists were with him. Thirty thousand feet above Africa, a reporter asked about the AIDS epidemic devouring the continent. Standing in the aisle by the flight map, the Pope replied that money alone was not the answer. He added, "If there is no human dimension, if Africans do not help by responsible behavior, the problem cannot be overcome by the distribution of prophylactics. On the contrary, they increase it."

World response was swift and caustic. The *New York Times* said he "deserves no credence when he distorts scientific findings about the value of condoms in slowing the spread of the AIDS virus." The *Washington Post* declared: "Pope Benedict XVI is wrong" because "the evidence says so." The top medical journal *The Lancet*, not given to hyperbole, called his comments "outrageous and wildly inaccurate." And multinational organizations and entire governments throughout Europe passed consensus statements and even legislation vilifying the Pope.

Yet he was right about *Africa*. And soon I got the opportunity to jump into this bedlam by saying so. As director of the Harvard AIDS Prevention Research Project and senior research scientist at the Harvard School of Public Health, I received a call from a writer at a prominent national magazine who asked straight out about the ruckus. I hesitated at first. I knew that if I said the Pope had articulated the solution better than *The Lancet*, I would be inviting trouble. Condom distribution has helped in some places. It just hasn't worked in Africa, where two of every three AIDS victims live today. And the Pope opposes condom use *period*, while I support it as a backup and even as a primary prevention strategy in some countries.

On Shepherd One the Pope does not answer questions off-the-cuff, like a politician at a news conference. Instead, reporters submit queries in advance and he mulls them over before deciding which ones to answer and how. And he had said: condom distribution will worsen the problem. Not condoms, but condom *distribution*, as a program. And not just condom distribution, but condom distribution *without responsible sexual behavior*. He had summarized the best current research on AIDS prevention in Africa.

In 1988, I first advocated the inexpensive, commonsense strategies I have fought for ever since. Millions of men and women would still be alive in Africa if we had followed them. But what I call "AIDS World" took a different path, and the best and the brightest in medicine and public health have led us to a global disaster of epic proportions. In fact, we are now experiencing the greatest avoidable epidemic in history. HIV has infected some forty-six million people in Africa and about eighteen million have died. That's equivalent to Hiroshima about ninety times over. Incidentally, the term "AIDS World" was inspired by journalist Maureen Dowd's book about an alternate universe called *Bushworld* ("It's their reality. We just live and die in it").[1]

The results are visible in urban neighborhoods like Soweto, in Johannesburg. On weekends there, police struggle to keep funeral processions from causing gridlock. At the crammed cemeteries dirges from nearby services compete for mourners' ears. Beyond the graveyards in Africa, twelve million AIDS orphans scramble to survive. Many have moved into tiny shacks with relatives who can hardly afford to feed them, or have become heads of their own threadbare households. Other orphans wander the streets homeless and malnourished. In some African countries AIDS patients fill half the hospital beds. In children's AIDS wards there is the eerie hush of babies too weak to cry. The disease is honeycombing societies and impoverishing nations for decades to come. And we—global AIDS programs—have ignored the prevention methods that help while wasting billions on strategies that don't. In human terms this is the most important health story of our generation.

The Pope was essentially taking a moral stance—that's what popes do—and I knew I would be risking further career damage if I publicly agreed with him. I would be saying that *The Lancet*, major agencies, and highly respected newspapers understood the epidemiological bottom line less than this religious leader. I could expect harsh attacks, and as a result I might lose some credibility, weaken my future impact on AIDS discussions, and harm my efforts to stop the spread of AIDS itself. I had worked in this field long enough to know the game. There were other places to speak out. I didn't have to do it here, in support of the Pope.

I'd noticed that the Pope hadn't used that great conversation stopper: "abstinence." Rather, he had stressed *faithfulness*. I realized that the platform of a national magazine could let me skewer enduring myths and force the world's attention on the fact that AIDS is different in Africa. When I talk about "African AIDS," I'm referring to the worst epidemics on earth (sometimes called hyperepidemics), found in about a dozen African countries with prevalence rates of more than 5 percent. Condom use doesn't work here, for important reasons, yet most "experts" have yet to acknowledge this research and simply assume that noncondom programs lead to mass deaths. As a result, we have seen mass deaths in Africans, unnecessarily and for too long.

These factors didn't all flash through my mind, however. The brain is nimble and weighs them just below conscious awareness. I had only seconds to decide how—or whether—to answer the reporter's question. So I told her that the best science actually supports the Pope's comment. In fact, it shows that condom use in Africa often correlates with an *increase* in HIV, just as he had said, and that "responsible" behavior—fidelity in particular—is beyond question much of the solution. (Male circumcision is the other key factor.) Fidelity is not abstinence. It is sex with one person, not sex with no one. The distinction may seem obvious, but it has repeatedly eluded policymakers. Largely on the basis of this interview, at least 250 Internet articles and blog discussions erupted within weeks, with such headlines as "Harvard AIDS Expert Says Pope Is Correct." I was soon speaking to radio interviewers on CBS, the BBC, and Sirius-XM, from such countries as Brazil, Canada, Italy, Peru, Spain, and Ukraine. I did numerous online interviews with both Catholic and secular news media, and I appeared on a national television show.

I also published an op-ed in the *Washington Post* on March 29, 2009, which intensified the debate.[2] Several other newspapers ran my piece in full. Hundreds of other papers quoted parts of it, as did literally thousands of bloggers. More interviews ensued. Some reporters were incredulous, apparently convinced that I was serving up conservative balderdash. For instance, William Crawley, from the BBC in Northern Ireland, informed me that UNAIDS and other organizations had all agreed that condoms were the "best weapon" we had against AIDS. He seemed amazed at my response: "I would be very careful about trusting the UNAIDS organization for anything scientific, anything having to do with, for example, statistics about AIDS. They have had to backpedal and retract a lot of their basic statistics. It may seem pretty shocking for somebody like me to disagree with UNAIDS, but the fact is that UNAIDS is changing its thinking on this matter."[3]

In fact, UNAIDS was just about to release a report on southern Africa more or less agreeing with me and the Pope. But Crawley plainly didn't believe me, and it wasn't his fault. He was just being a good, skeptical journalist, and he had heard otherwise for too long. The chasm between general opinion and scientific truth is so wide that one side is barely visible from the other, and UNAIDS itself has been partly responsible. Anyone can read its admission of statistical errors on its Web site—and if only its distortions had ended there.[4] As I tried to explain the evidence, commentators kept referring to UNAIDS as *the* authority. So I chuckled when I read a comment about me on a heated blog discussion: "Just because someone from Harvard says something, it doesn't make it true. You're committing the fallacy of an appeal to authority."

Why did this media uproar occur? Why did UNAIDS have its facts so wrong for so long? And how could the Pope take *The Lancet* to school on a hyperepidemic?

On September 6, 2006, I testified before a House subcommittee about fidelity and abstinence (or delay of age of first sexual intercourse), the most effective approach we knew of in Africa. Opponents had tagged it "abstinence-only," however, and it had become the quarry in a political foxhunt. Indeed, Rep. Barbara Lee (D-CA) had introduced legislation to repeal its funding, and she led the charge against me. "The rest of the world, quite frankly, disagrees with what you're saying, Dr. Green," she stated. "The rest of the world *gets it.*" In other words, why wasn't I on the bus? My answer was, Who would want to be on this bus? It's gone off a cliff, and its wheels are spinning.

I told Representative Lee that repealing fidelity-abstinence would be a gift to the disease. It would pat the HIV virus on the shoulder and say, Go forth and multiply! Most of the AIDS catastrophe had been preventable, I explained, and then I described the strategy in Uganda. Uganda's fidelity-abstinence program had cut its AIDS rate by two-thirds, from 15 percent to 5 percent between 1991 and 2004. This effort alone might have saved hundreds of thousands of lives. It was the greatest triumph against AIDS in history—and its price tag fit African national budgets. During the early years it had cost about twenty-five cents annually per person.

The campaign in Uganda had brought about most behavior change in the late 1980s and the early 1990s, before condoms were widely available. Then Western advisers arrived, heavily promoted these devices, and began undoing the program. I told the subcommittee that today the infection rate in Uganda was rising again.

But soon I was wondering why they called it a "hearing," because no one was listening. By the end of it, Representative Lee had promised not to rest until she had abolished the funding for fidelity-abstinence.

A few months later I ran into Barbara Lee at a rally to defeat this earmark, in the U.S. Congress building. Population Action International, for whom I had once consulted, had organized the rally, and my former colleagues in family planning warmly welcomed me. I asked Representative Lee if I could meet with her to show her important data about AIDS in Africa. She agreed. But when it came to scheduling, she seemed busier than Ben Bernanke during the meltdown. It made me think of the *New Yorker* cartoon: "Let's see . . . Thursday's not good for me . . . or Friday . . . How about never? Is *never* good for you?"

In 2007, Representative Lee introduced a bill to fight AIDS in Africa by supporting, among other measures, microenterprise and job-training programs, education, property and inheritance rights, and equal rights for women. These are excellent goals, but they have eluded foreign-aid efforts for decades. Even if we somehow attained them, most of these goals would have no impact on African AIDS prevention. Rep. Barbara Lee is actually one of the good guys. She really cares about AIDS. I admire and respect her for spurning money from certain pernicious lobbying groups.

Most AIDS policymakers mean well, and many are (or were) good friends of mine. But given the dire consequences, we must understand why they have erred. When the ancient astronomer Ptolemy said the sun orbits the earth, he made one of the most notorious mistakes in scientific history, yet no one *died* from it. But when Westerners convinced Botswana that condoms would stop AIDS, the results were catastrophic. About one in five adults there now has HIV.

I first went to Africa in 1977, and I have since visited some twenty countries throughout the continent. I have talked to people in the cities and the hinterland, in the chambers of power, and in the villages and homesteads. I have met with poor and remote people beyond the peripheral vision of policymakers. I have listened and learned. AIDS is different in Africa. In most places AIDS primarily attacks special populations at chronic high risk, like gay men and injecting drug users (IDUs), and HIV rates remain comparatively low in overall populations. But AIDS has ravaged whole nations in parts of sub-Saharan Africa, and it spreads primarily by heterosexual intercourse. So it's critical to understand the sexual, marital, and other behaviors and values of Africans. Yet Western planners have designed AIDS prevention in Africa as if it were just like the rest of the world, at least until very recently.

A Zambian doctor once asked me, "Why are there no AIDS programs for most of us? Why are they all just for high-risk groups, like prostitutes or drug addicts?" One reason is that the official communication channels shrank to pinholes when researchers offered the fidelity evidence. I quoted this doctor and others like her in one of several reports the U.S. government commissioned me to write but then decided not to release. By the early 2000s I would meet a few other AIDS researchers with impeccable credentials whose data also pointed to the success of fidelity promotion in Africa and the failure of condoms. These scientists were also having great difficulty getting published.

So myths have circulated. At the anti–abstinence-fidelity rally mentioned earlier, Rep. Chris Shays (R-CT) said that "asking an African to abstain is like trying to repeal the law of gravity" and that "abstinence-only is ignorance-only." The first line echoes the nineteenth-century colonialists; the second is ignorance itself. I must forever remind myself: Guys like him are only repeating what they think science has demonstrated. They mean well. Yet their beliefs affect life and death in Africa.

Here are some persisting myths about AIDS in Africa:

· HIV infection rates are still increasing.
· We can't prevent AIDS effectively unless we make antiretroviral drug treatment available.
· We can't prevent AIDS effectively unless people are tested and know their HIV status.
· Condoms will prevent AIDS, at least if we can persuade people to use them.
· At least some condom use is better than no condom use. At least condom promotion can't hurt.
· Most African teens are already having sex.
· Most Africans have far more sex partners than Westerners do.
· Promotion of abstinence is not realistic because (African) men cannot abstain from sex.
· Promotion of fidelity is not realistic because (African) men cannot be faithful.
· Africans are the most promiscuous people in the world.
· Marriage is dangerous because husbands infect their wives with HIV.
· Poverty drives AIDS epidemics.
· Gender imbalance drives AIDS epidemics.

- Lack of education drives AIDS epidemics.
- Civil war and civil strife in general drive AIDS epidemics.
- African women are powerless.
- Use of fear messages to change behavior is counterproductive.
- Sexual behavior does not and cannot be changed.

The list could go on. It is often easier to say, "Whatever you think you know about AIDS is wrong when it comes to Africa." Because whatever elements of truth *some* of these statements might have for *some* countries, *none of them is true for Africa*. Several of them are the perfect opposites of the truth. For example, HIV rates tend to *increase* with higher levels of education, income, and condom use. In fact, no one has ever proved any positive impact on national or population-wide HIV infection rates on AIDS in Africa from standard, Western-style interventions. These include not just condom promotion but treatment of sexually transmitted infections, voluntary counseling and testing, diaphragm use, microbicides, "safer sex" counseling, vaccines, and income generation. Yet we have aggressively pushed many of these strategies, and poured money into researching the others. I have been using this list of myths since 2006 or earlier. As this book went to press in the fall of 2010, UNAIDS startled many people with its 2010 report that announced: "22 of the most affected countries in sub-Saharan Africa have reduced HIV incidence by more than 25%." Of course, it assumes increased condom use is a major cause.

Uganda is not the only nation in Africa where we have undermined a successful program. When Kenya developed a similar fidelity campaign—called One Man, One Woman—Western activists expressed outrage at this "narrow" concept of marriage. I myself have witnessed U.S. bullying of AIDS programs in Zambia. One person told me that if I ever described the incident in print, I would never work for the government again. This book will test that forecast.

Ironically, the Ugandan approach we've dismissed could be just what we need to cut AIDS among gay men and IDUs back home. Behavior-change programs have slashed nicotine dependency in the United States, for instance, and could increase fidelity among gay men and drug abstention (or at least needle avoidance) among addicts as well. Such primary prevention should be the foundation of all disease-control efforts. Yet special interest groups have brought great pressure on funders of billion-dollar programs to exempt AIDS from the normal rules of medicine and public health. This phenomenon is called "AIDS exceptionalism." Its consequences show why the rules existed in the first place.

In 2003, I wrote *Rethinking AIDS Prevention*, which explained the Uganda story in detail.[5] To my surprise, the book had a rather serious impact. I was appointed to the President's Advisory Council on HIV/AIDS. But this was the Bush administration, and I was fairly naive about the fierce culture wars I was stumbling into. The Bush people were already on the side of "abstinence," but not because of data from Africa (or perhaps anywhere). On the other hand, some gay scholars had written that the very word "monogamy" offended them. Speeches and congressional testimony based on drafts of my book had helped get the earmark for fidelity-abstinence—the one Representative Lee had disliked so much—into President Bush's 2003 fifteen-billion-dollar bill to fight AIDS globally. Then a worldwide backlash ensued. How could anyone publicly oppose fidelity? I was about to find out.

For the record I am a lifelong, outspoken liberal-progressive-leftist. I have never voted for a Republican. I would have cast my ballot for Ralph Nader in two recent presidential elections if he hadn't been siphoning votes from the Democrats in two tight races. I have always supported reproductive rights and sexual freedom, and I spent many years working in contraception, family planning, and condom marketing. I am not an active adherent of any sect, denomination, or religion. I shouldn't have to say these things, but such is the level of argument that some people judge one's findings by one's politics and vice versa. Of course, that isn't science at all; it's ideology.

I believe that truth eventually prevails, whether it arrives with a fanfare or claws its way out of an iron box at the bottom of the sea. And the truth is finally, slowly, starting to prevail in Africa. The two countries with the worst HIV epidemics, Swaziland and Botswana, have launched fidelity campaigns. More research supporting fidelity is appearing in the relevant journals. Conferences on the strategy are occurring both in the United States and abroad. Even UNAIDS has stated, at least in one regional 2009 report, that fidelity deserves higher priority than condom promotion.[6]

Meanwhile, under pressure from the Great Recession, the West has begun to cut off funds for the antiretroviral drugs that have kept African AIDS victims alive. Many more millions who should never have gotten ill in the first place may die of the disease in the coming years. Ultimately we must ask these fundamental questions: Why has the spread and prevention of AIDS in Africa differed so dramatically from AIDS in most other places? Why have we poured billions into prevention programs that don't work? And how could we possibly have committed these genocide-level mistakes? This book attempts to answer these questions and reveal the inside story behind one of the tragic blunders in modern history. For those who only want to focus on the empirical evidence, see my book coauthored by Allison Herling Ruark, *AIDS Behavior and Culture: Understanding Evidence-based Prevention*.[7]

PART I

THE ROAD TO FIDELITY

Dissent is the native activity of the scientist.

JACOB BRONOWSKI
Science and Human Values

CHAPTER 1

Gangs, Maroons, and the Egg Taboo

Before Africa, there was an illegal trip upriver in Suriname. Before Harvard, there were the Sewer Rats. Before congressional subcommittees, there were long talks with African spirit mediums. These activities may seem irrelevant to spotting the fidelity solution and promoting it as the means to combating the spread of AIDS, but some of these activities were crucial and partly explain why others took longer.

I was born at the start of the Boomer generation that came of age in the 1960s. I grew up in a liberal family, and I still have photos of my mother with Robert Kennedy and Hubert Humphrey. My father, Marshall Green, was a career foreign service officer who rose to become a much respected ambassador, assistant secretary of state, and then a leading family-planning advocate and authority. When he died, my brother and I got a condolence cable from Henry Kissinger, who was forever grateful that my father had omitted from his memoir certain stories about Nixon's trip to China and a world-class blunder Kissinger almost caused.

Because of my father's career, my family often moved. I have fine childhood memories of New Zealand and Sweden. Later, in Washington D.C., I distinguished the family escutcheon by cofounding the Sewer Rats gang. We had black leather jackets with our names on the back, Elvis haircuts—the works. I began smoking (only tobacco in those days) at age twelve, got a police record for a switchblade incident of which I was most proud, and experienced the sweet taste of rebellion. Why I was the black sheep of the family I cannot say.

Starting at age ten, I attended two boarding schools for almost five years: Fay School, where actor Peter Fonda was as miserable as I was, and super-elite Groton, where my father and Franklin Roosevelt had thrived, and which I hated. The feeling was reciprocal. After I had been expelled for a "chronic negative attitude" toward authority, my mother informed me that my life was over. One bitterly cold day in January 1960, we moved to Seoul, Korea, and I enrolled at the American high school for military brats. There I disproved my mother's dictum by cofounding the Aborigines gang and losing my virginity amid heavy drinking and wild times. I resumed my hoodlum life and started a rock-and-roll band. We played at local nightclubs and got paid partly in booze.

One day my history teacher, Mr. Hervey, caught me looking at someone else's paper during a quiz. He confronted me and asked me if I'd like to be handed over to the principal. In a mock-indignant voice I asked him if he were man enough to step outside with me. He backed down and I felt lousy almost at once. Yet a few months later, I was surprised and rather touched when he shyly asked me if he could play his tenor sax with us at a school dance on the '50s hit "Tequila." A photo of this strange rapprochement recently surfaced on the Internet.

I became the first kid in my 11th grade to get a "social" disease. I soon discovered that girls in my school were not quite as thrilled as guys about my accumulating triumphs. Still, promiscuity was the name of the game and I was clearly an all-star. In my high school yearbook for the Class of '62, the prophecy for me was: "Shot by a jealous husband." Friends from this earlier life (including my ex-wife, who left me because of my infidelity) can hardly believe Ted Green promotes faithfulness these days.

I surprised my parents by entirely skipping my sophomore year.

They might have been even more surprised if they'd known how I'd managed it. I happened to be in a taxi with our Korean band manager, who also worked at the high school. He had gotten a call asking him to drop everything and pick up our school principal, who was in a brothel, robbed of his money and clothes. I waited a discreet week and then went to see the principal about moving ahead one year. He decided that some courses I had taken at Groton could be considered high-school level, therefore I had earned enough credits to leap ahead a year. No mention of the previous encounter.

In other words, you won't find my picture if you look up "prude" in the dictionary. And—as perhaps you have surmised—I have a problem with authority. I dislike it, probably more than most people, as shown by my expulsions from Groton, from summer camp, and eventually from Harvard's Center for Population Studies (even as I write this book). I like to stick up for the weak and stick it to the rich and powerful, especially if they are arrogant. Whether my joy in puncturing these floating, self-important bags of professionalism is a bias to overcome, a form of masochism, or a useful analytic tool, I wish at least to be forthright about it.

Two powerful forces shaped my life. The first was rebellion. My parents had laid out a Life Plan for Son #2 and it differed little from that for Son #1, my well-behaved elder brother: Groton, Yale, then one or more graduate degrees, whereupon noblesse oblige nudged us away from Wall Street ("Making money is so *vulgar*," my mother used to say) and toward the foreign service, an Ivy League professorship, or an Episcopal bishophood. We descend directly from the first Episcopal bishop of the United States, Samuel Seabury, who gazed down on us from the often-invoked family pantheon, along with five colonial governors. So to become my own person, I had to spurn all of the above and become a juvenile delinquent, as every logician and psychologist would agree.

The second force that shaped my life was yearning toward achievement. For all was not right with my alternative life. My mother had drummed into my head that I was a failure and would always be a failure. Not like my peerless older brother. Part of me needed to prove my mother wrong. I could be as good as my older brother—if I cared to. I just didn't. But what if I changed my mind later on? I realized I shouldn't cut off my options entirely. So the whole time I was a hoodlum, and later a hippie and druggie, I was also quietly working on a degree or a postdoc or writing an article or a book. Most of my friends didn't know about that secret life.

The Vietnam War fed into this dualism. As tens of thousands of people in my generation died overseas and the question "Why are we in Vietnam?" stumped the officials who had started the war (including my father, then assistant secretary of state for East Asian affairs), I spent my time doing antiwar activism and, to tell the truth, getting high a lot. When LBJ tried to draft me in 1966, I trotted out my juvie police record in the preinduction exam. They asked if I was rehabilitated, and I said, "Hell no." They informed me I *had* to be, because it said right there on paper that I had a master's degree. In the end I became a conscientious objector and performed alternative service in an all-black psychiatric ward at a D.C. mental hospital. I also served as draft counselor and wrote a column for war objectors. With my press pass I got front-row seats—once right next to peace activists Jane Fonda and Shirley MacLaine—at major antiwar events.

Meanwhile, in college at George Washington University, I was leaning toward clinical psychology, through which I hoped to gain insights into why I felt generally alienated from the human race. But before long I discovered an entire academic field of study—a *profession*—peopled by the alienated: anthropology. The literary theorist Susan Sontag had recently published an enticing essay called "The Anthropologist as Hero" about the heroic journey into the unknown that anthropologists take.[1] Professors in this field wore dusty cowboy boots, offered courses in arcane subjects like "Magic, Witchcraft, and Religion," opposed the Vietnam War, and smoked pot with their followers. It was hard to resist.

I remained in anthropology through a master's degree and a Ph.D. because it seemed intrinsically interesting. I looked forward to total-immersion fieldwork in an exotic culture, billed by the likes of American anthropologist A. L. Kroeber as an experience far more transformative than long-term psychoanalysis. But I still had no real career goals. As a grad student in anthropology, at the age of twenty-six, I set off for the South American rain forest.

Among the Maroons

I arrived in 1971 with my young wife, a one-year-old son, and our trusty mixed German shepherd Karl (he preferred the Marxist spelling) in the capital of Suriname, Paramaribo, which sprawled along the piranha-filled Suriname River. It was still a Dutch colony and would remain so until 1975. I intended to voyage deep into the jungle to examine the impact of Dutch colonial culture on the fragile matrilineal kinship system of the Matawai. I felt privileged to be about to investigate a never-before studied tribe in the tropics, just like Margaret Mead (about whom more anon). It was an opportunity from a bygone era.

The Matawai fascinated me. They were Maroons—that is, people descended from the three hundred thousand African slaves the Dutch had shipped over to work, sweat, and die in the sugar, coffee, and cocoa plantations. Their lives had been dreadful even by slave standards. However forbidding the rain forest, it had sucked them in by the thousands. (Hence the name "Maroons," which originally referred to domesticated animals that ran off and became wild.) When owners recaptured these slaves, they had them drawn and quartered, and hung the dismembered carcasses up on trees to discourage other slaves from flight.

The Maroons did not ignore this message. They attacked the plantations at night, freeing more slaves—including women. Soon they established "rebel societies" in the Amazon forest and developed a Creole language based on Portuguese, English, and various Afri-can tongues, sprinkled with Yiddish words (some plantation owners were Jews who had originally come from Brazil). After years of war with the Dutch, the Maroons signed a treaty that secured their inde-pendence in 1760. Thus, twenty-three years before the U.S. Revolu-tionary War ended, they became the first people in the Americas to win freedom from Europe. When I was in Suriname, the colonial government still paid tribute to the Maroons in the form of rum, machetes, pots, and pans in return for their remaining peaceful and not incinerating plantations.

All in all, this was just the right place for a nonconformist like me with serious authority issues. It sure beat fighting a misbegotten war half a world away. I was eager to go upriver and start fieldwork. But I had a problem. I needed to obtain formal permission from the host country to do research in tribal areas. In Paramaribo I made contact with the Matawai at a little slum building where Amerindians and Maroons from the interior could hang their hammocks, sleep, and cook during their short trips to town. On my first visit there, I met an American woman, a Ph.D. linguist, whose goal was to learn the lan-guage of the Saramakas, the tribe one river over from the Matawai. She had been waiting for formal government approval for two years. The closest she ever came to her tribe was this part of town.

Yikes! I had only two years for my entire project.

So I went up the river with my wife, son, and dog. I simply showed up among the Matawai and began doing fieldwork. And there, day by day, I waited for someone in the government to kick me out.

I hardly expected air-conditioning and featherbeds in the jungle, but life there proved far more challenging than I'd imagined, what with killer parasites, poisonous snakes, flesh-stripping piranhas, clouds of predatory mosquitoes, vampire bats, culture shock, and broken communication in an unwritten language. My wife got a bad case of typhoid fever, and overall I realized that I'd had a laughably shallow understanding of the word "inconvenience."

At first the Matawai thought I was a missionary who was pretending for some reason to not be one. Who else but a man of the Bible would come to live with strangers under these harsh conditions, especially with a wife and child? After I learned enough Matawai to converse, they tried a few scatological, missionary-busting songs in my presence. When I laughed in the right places, they figured, "This guy must be OK. We don't need to worry about what we say in his presence." In fact, they eventually became proud to have their own white family in their midst. Soon people were bringing me things to fix, like wristwatches and outboard motors. I tried to explain what a klutz was, but they insisted: "Aren't these things made by white people? Are you not white? Please repair!"

My wife and I came to greatly admire the Maroons, the first non-Western people I came to know really well. I have a little Dutch ancestry in my blueblood lineage, so it's possible my ancestors enslaved, tortured, and killed the ancestors of these Matawai. Yet they adopted us and treated us with the utmost hospitality. Although I proved a letdown with Paleface gadgetry, I came to see how we provided comic relief from the tedium of the *tristes tropiques*. Picture me in a loincloth and toga, seated with the elders at an all-night festival. The village chief would challenge other men in their twenties to name all the villages in Matawai territory, whether existing or abandoned, over the past two centuries. Men my age were learning about the outside world, via radio and trips to town, and some found the Motown sound much more worthy of attention than vanished villages. If someone failed the history test, an elder would say, "Ha! Now listen to the Curious One. He can name them all!"

In fact, I came to see that as someone intrigued by the Old Ways, I was a conservative in my adopted society yet a radical revolutionary in my own. After that epiphany I could never take political classifications as seriously as most people do. I learned something even more important. When anthropologists study an exotic culture, we practice something called cultural relativism, meaning we don't superimpose our own moral or other judgments on the culture. For example, we do not say, "The tribe I lived with practiced a primitive, anti-Christian practice that demeans and disempowers women." Instead, we suspend our values and simply describe what we see. That is what I learned to do with the Matawai, and that is what I have done ever since in my professional life.

This approach is scientific—we describe what *is* rather than what *should be* in our own highly important opinion—but it has a second virtue too: clarity. It forces our eyes open. When we dismiss a practice as immoral, we often see its details less precisely and its function not at all. This blurring happens automatically, and most of us are scarcely aware of it. Frankly, I didn't think too much about it at the time either. But later in my career I would think about this idea a lot.

About six months after our arrival in Suriname, government officials appeared at the village of the Paramount Chief for a formal annual tribute meeting. This was the pro forma giving of pots and machetes to keep the plantations unburned. I watched the government guys carefully. Would they send me to jail, or at least research limbo? They were also watching me, a strange white guy sitting with the council of elders. I had become an honorary elder, despite my youth, because I had shown proper respect for the Old Ways. These government men didn't confront me, but before they left that day, they asked the Paramount Chief what I was doing in his village. The chief replied, "No problem. This is the Curious One, whom we've adopted, and who is currently providing labor in the planting fields of his adopted grandmother-in-law, living as a good Matawai." Because tribes enjoyed a fair amount of autonomy before independence, that did the trick. No permission needed. I had proved myself with my research subjects and thereby avoided an endless dawdle in the capital.

After nearly two years of classical immersion-type ethnographic fieldwork (which anthropologists practice far less often nowadays), I was fluent in Matawai, a language spoken by two thousand souls and my ex-wife. I had had out-of-body mystical experiences with these people and become the adopted nephew of the Paramount Chief. I fully appreciated the complexities of a matrilineal kinship system under assault by the bilateral alternative of Dutch kinship. I was ready to tackle the world.

Alas, there was no great demand for matrilineal kinship-in-transition experts in 1973, nor was any boom anticipated. I spent my dissertation-writing year, as well as the next four, in temporary academic appointments, teaching introductory anthropology to large, unruly sections of lower classes and dreaming up new ways to interpret my dissertation material for publications in scholarly journals. More than once during a two-year appointment at West Virginia University, my department chair, Russ Bernard, suggested that I might find more satisfaction in applying anthropology to the problems of developing countries than in spinning out articles on the fission of matrilineal kinship groups facing detribalization.

But I resisted. I was a purist. I saw myself as seeking knowledge for its own sake. Practical applications were for Mr. Fix-Its rather than explorers, for engineers rather than scientists. Besides, the prospect daunted me. How could a person even begin to apply anthropology out there in the Real World? I mean, did I really know anything useful?

Epiphanies in a Famine

In the summer of 1977, I unexpectedly had an opportunity to visit five countries in the African Sahel, the semiarid fringe of the Sahara, to help evaluate population programs. This part of Africa had suffered a relentless drought for years. The desert was eating up the grasslands, and millions were starving. I felt I had been around a bit up to then, but I had never before seen babies wrinkled from dehydration or blank-eyed from rib-exposing marasmus.

In Niger I had a revelation. An officer with the United States

Agency for International Development (USAID) had commented to me: "You know, we have a terrible malnutrition problem among pregnant women, meaning their babies are born underweight and vulnerable. We have one good source of protein—eggs—but there's a taboo against pregnant women eating eggs. Now, if we could just figure out how to get around that taboo." I thought: *I could be doing that!* In a moment of illumination I saw that anthropology really could relieve suffering and save lives. Scholarly papers on the mysteries of matrilineal kinship were not the way. Large donor organizations were on the scene, but the more I spoke with people in their health and nutrition programs, the more I grew convinced that anthropology was a critical missing piece in their strategy. How could foreigners change the behavior of tribal and peasant peoples when they didn't understand it, much less the beliefs, values, attitudes, and indigenous knowledge systems that shaped it?

It is terribly easy to misunderstand Africa. For instance, whatever romanticized, counterculture ideas I had about African sexuality quickly vanished in the Sahel. I learned that sexual intercourse is a potent force in African culture, because it can result in pregnancy and thereby determine one's social identity—that is, what family, lineage, and clan a person belongs to, or whether he or she is socially recognized, legitimate. Moreover, intercourse involves the commingling of the powerful and potentially dangerous fluids of males and females. For these and other reasons, rules, norms, and customary laws always govern sexual relations.

Later in the trip, I had a second moment of illumination. I was at a cocktail party in Ghana when I ran into Michael Warren, a medical anthropologist from Iowa State University. He was setting up one of the first serious programs to work with traditional healers (the term they themselves prefer) on aspects of Western public health. About 80 percent of all people in sub-Saharan Africa rely on these healers for medical diagnosis and treatment, even if many also visit clinics. Traditional healers are thus the de facto primary health-care providers. Mike was teaching them to use oral rehydration salts on infants with diarrheal diseases, which are major baby-killers in Africa and beyond. This was clearly a program with life-or-death impact. I realized I could be applying my knowledge to issues on a grand scale, instead of teaching it to students fulfilling a social science requirement. So I made the decision: I would become an applied anthropologist. I have never regretted it.

A few years ago, after a fascinating three-hour interview with South African albinos, I persuaded my sweet, speed-typing wife Suzie to help me compile a list of other unusual people I have talked to over the years (usually with her at my side, smiling and showing that my intentions were peaceful). Here are some of the groups I have met and interviewed along the way:

- South African Albinism Society members
- Javanese transvestites
- Naxi (Chinese Himalayan) tribal healers
- Gypsies in the Montenegro mountains
- Prostitutes in Cambodia, China, Guyana, Indonesia, Philippines, Thailand, and elsewhere
- Guyanese male prostitutes and transvestites
- Palestinian refugees in Jordan
- Women with breast cancer in a Ukrainian hospital in Odessa
- Thyroid cancer victims from Chernobyl, Ukraine
- Christian and Muslim faith healers throughout Africa
- Spirit-possessed healers throughout Africa
- Carib Indians in the Amazon rain forest
- Injecting drug addicts in the Central Philippines
- Chinese drug addicts
- Palestinian victims of domestic abuse
- Bedouin refugees in the Gaza Strip
- Chakma tribesmen along the Bangladesh-Burmese border
- Escaped child soldiers from Angola and Mozambique

- Polish parliamentarians
- Rwandan Catholic leaders
- U.S. White House domestic policy advisers
- U.S. Senate and House Foreign Affairs and other committee members
- Forest Peoples' Fund for Conservation members in Suriname
- Russian narcologists (addiction specialists)
- American Indian recovering alcoholics in the Seattle area
- Hindu faith healers in Bangladesh
- Buddhist monks in northern Thailand
- Midwives in Upper Volta and Senegal
- Chiefs and princesses in the Kingdom of Swaziland
- African-American gay HIV-positive men in New Orleans
- Cuban veterans of African wars, in Cuba
- Catholic educators in Uganda
- Disabled orphans throughout Vietnam
- Veterans of the "American War" in Vietnam
- Christian faith healers in the Dominican Republic
- Film and TV censors of apartheid South Africa
- Sudanese mycologists (snail scientists)

And the list could go on. I have gained *ondofeni foe libi*, or what the Maroons call "Great Life Experience." Looking back, I probably had the best career possible for a guy with hair-trigger authority issues—"best" in terms of personal growth and enrichment, enjoyment, travel, independence, and gathering material for publications. Do they call that stumbling into bliss?

I never could have dreamed up this kind of life. I didn't even know such careers existed. Yet mine almost ended before it began.

CHAPTER 2

The Visitation

The United States Agency for International Development (USAID) is one of the most important presences in the developing world, because it dispenses most U.S. nonmilitary foreign aid. Ned Greeley, an anthropologist friend of mine from grad school, helped me get my first consulting gig with that agency in Sudan in 1980. He went on to have a long and fruitful career with USAID, but this two-week assignment almost ended my career.

Before I went to Africa this time, I worried: *What don't I know about Sudan? The culture? The history? The disease patterns? What might I miss?* I have now been to the continent countless times and I still have those concerns. Yet most Americans I work with in Africa seem brimming with confidence. Maybe engineers and agricultural economists feel their skills need no adjustment anywhere on earth. But overall I suspect that grave self-doubt is the proper attitude when arriving in Africa with nothing but the boon of American wisdom. However, these anxieties had nothing to do with my near-termination. I wrote an irreverent diary about this first job, just to amuse my colleagues. It wound up published in a major journal and a U.S. official I had lampooned threatened a lawsuit.

Narrowly escaping termination of my brand-new life in applied anthropology, I managed to land a job as "social scientist" on the Rural Waterborne Disease Project in Swaziland in 1981. Swaziland is a landlocked kingdom about the size of New Jersey, surrounded on three sides by South Africa and the fourth by Mozambique. It is the last true monarchy in Africa, yet unlike most governments on the continent, Swaziland is neither a despotism nor a kleptocracy. Rather, it operates under a system of "representative polygamy," in which the Swazi ruler takes a wife from each major kingdom and clan, and thus keeps the peace. Indeed, for more than a century there have been no wars, no coups d'état, and none of the horrors many Africans have had to endure.

Once in Swaziland, I quickly strayed beyond my mandate and began hobnobbing with the traditional healers. It happened that another USAID-funded project wanted someone to do a quick study of these healers as potential partners in public-health ventures, such as getting kids with diarrheal diseases to drink oral rehydration salts. I took on the added responsibility—and suddenly I was like Michael Warren, working directly with the healers.

I also met Joe G., who quickly became my translator, key informant, "culture broker," and co-investigator. As a reporter, he was skilled at interviewing. If African nations allowed them to operate in their countries, he would have been an investigative journalist—my kind of guy: get the story right and damn the authorities. Joe had the highly useful talent of putting people at ease and getting them to speak freely. Princes in Swaziland do not necessarily open up and spill the beans to commoners. He and I shared a fascination with spirit mediums (*sangomas*) and the possibility that people (maybe even ourselves) might acquire supernatural powers. I remember the time Joe and I got up at 4 a.m. to try to glimpse the *tinzunzu* water spirits, translucent beings alleged to rise just before dawn from the foamy rapids of the Mbuluzi River to greet newly initiated spirit mediums. A *gobela*, a ritual specialist, had to invite you to the occasion, and we'd gotten lucky. Alas, the spirits didn't appear that day, we were told, because someone had skipped or misperformed some fragment of the ritual.

I left Swaziland in 1985, but I kept getting research assignments that brought me back there for a few weeks at a time. Joe always dropped whatever he was doing to help me in my research. Once we interviewed executives of several leading businesses in an industrial park. Joe was sure one general manager, who kept late hours, was a zombie—one of those uncanny, silent, resurrected corpses who became slaves to their revivers and who, reports said, often tilled their owners' fields after dark, weirdly sweatless no matter how hard the toil. Joe and I had tried but failed to find a zombie one night when we were driving back from Durban, South Africa. He and I had many unforgettable adventures, and he would become my best friend in Africa.

Meanwhile, I began working directly with USAID, helping it find ways to collaborate with traditional healers in the Swazi public health-care system. We did a survey and found that nearly 99 percent of healers wanted to learn Western techniques and collaborate with doctors and nurses, a finding I would encounter elsewhere in Africa. I gave a presentation of our results to the medical association of Swaziland, thinking all these doctors would be happy that the traditional healers wanted to learn. After I finished, the questions came at me in a rush from the floor: *Why aren't these guys in jail? They're practicing medicine without a license! Why isn't someone arresting them?*

Despite this reception, we set up some workshops for the traditional healers. Together with my colleagues in the Swazi Ministry of Health, we developed an approach that consisted of workshops for the mutual exchange of medical and healing knowledge (we avoided the term "training" because we were also learning much from them). The first healers came in disguise, in civilian clothes, like priests scoring drugs. But by the second or third workshop, they were arriving in full regalia, all decked out in feathers and beads. They were about to face the biggest challenge of their lives. So was I.

Advent

In the early 1980s U.S. scientists first noticed a strange and scary medical condition. It seemed as deadly as dioxin, and its very nature was hard to grasp at first, because it used other diseases to kill. Doctors first recognized the condition through an illness previously almost unknown to the public: Kaposi's sarcoma. This rare and fairly mild cancer struck almost no one at the time but the elderly. However, in March 1981 a cluster of much more severe cases appeared, and the victims were young. The oddity set off warnings. Two months later, the Centers for Disease Control (CDC) reported that five men in Southern California had contracted Pneumocystis carinii pneumonia, another rarity. All these first patients in California and New York had been gay men.

In December 1981, UK specialists diagnosed the first clear case of a wasting disease that seemed to open the body to a world of infections and tumors. No treatment helped, and gay men seemed the sole sufferers. The ailment even resisted all proffered names (including "gay-related immune deficiency," or GRID), until July 1982 at a meeting in Washington, D.C., where the condition got one that stuck: Acquired Immune Deficiency Syndrome, or AIDS. Yet the acronym set it further apart, as if its horrors required an aseptic, bureaucratic label.

Its modus operandi remained bewildering, and the puzzle only grew as we learned more about it. By the end of 1982 the condition was appearing in transfusion recipients and children, proof that it was not just a gay disease. In 1983, Dr. Lawrence K. Altman wrote in the *New York Times:* "In many parts of the world there is anxiety, bafflement, a sense that something has to be done—although no one knows what."[1] The cause of AIDS was still unknown. In May of 1983 a French team led by Dr. Luc Montagnier announced it had isolated a new virus that might be the culprit. It received the name "lymphadenopathy-associated virus" (LAV). In 1984 an American team led by Dr. Robert Gallo isolated a virus and asserted it was the pathogen. He claimed priority and called it HTLV-3. One of the bitterest scientific dust-ups in recent memory ensued; the virus had no official name until 1986, when the International Committee on the Taxonomy of Viruses navigated around both contenders in favor of "human immunodeficiency virus," or HIV. But the French were clearly first, and on October 6, 2008, Montagnier and his colleague Francoise Barre-Sinoussi received the Nobel Prize for their work.

As people kept dying, we learned that the bug was a little ball of nastiness. Not only was it always fatal, but it worked by stealth. It could lurk in the body for a decade or more, silent but contagious, so oblivious victims could pass it on again and again. And it had an especially dangerous initial stage we would learn about only later. AIDS is a disease of the immune system, the apparatus that normally fights off disease. Think of it as an army that keeps a nation free from invasion. AIDS corrupts that army from within. It actually turns soldier cells—called helper T-cells—into zombies manufacturing HIV clones. These new clones eventually kill the soldiers and spread out. Over time the army grows so decimated that the body's other foes have easy pickings. Kaposi's sarcoma, for instance, thrives in young people whose immune systems would otherwise have scotched it.

HIV does have one weakness—fortunately, or the havoc would be hard to imagine: it doesn't spread easily. No one ever gets HIV by breathing or shaking a hand. HIV requires intimate contact, a mixing of body secretions, especially blood.

Much later we would learn how HIV came about, how long people have suffered from it, and why it had such a long latency period. Meanwhile, throughout the 1980s the disease was spreading through Africa at very different rates, and there its victims differed from those in the West. The risk factors then noted in American cases were homosexuality, intravenous drug use, and transfusions, and somehow there was a Haitian connection. But in late 1983 researchers in Rwanda found that a combination of city dwelling, reasonably high income, and heterosexual promiscuity could increase the risk.[2] In a 1984 study of twenty-three African AIDS patients, not one had any of the American risk factors; instead, the main vehicle seemed to be heterosexual sex.[3] AIDS had also appeared in Uganda, and studies in 1985 found that it, too, occurred mainly among promiscuous heterosexuals, people like my younger self. In other words, African AIDS looked poised to infect far more people.

Remarkably, the first effective means of controlling HIV arose almost before we knew what it was. Unlike other European countries, from 1983 through 1991, Holland conducted a public information campaign among Amsterdam gays promoting behavior change. They highlighted the dangers of anal sex—the primary transmission route for gay men—and the relative ineffectiveness of condoms. They used a two-tiered approach, urging abandonment of hazardous sex and condom use as a backup strategy. The message was: "Don't do anal sex. But if you do it anyway, use condoms."

The upshot? A large proportion of men ceased anal intercourse, which had only a recent history in the Dutch gay community anyway and is still not especially common in many places such as Asia.[4] The gay community there went back to sexual practices with a much, much lower risk of HIV infection. New cases of HIV fell quickly and significantly.[5] It was pretty straightforward: people could and would change their sexual behavior. Gay men moved away from high-risk behavior and had far fewer ongoing partnerships—and the rate of new infections fell. A similar, if less clearly documented, change actually occurred in America at this time: gay men had fewer sexual partners, motivated by fear of seeing friends sicken and die, and in response to actions such as the closing of gay bathhouses.[6]

So where are the scientific and journalistic spotlights? Where are the AIDS activists shouting and pointing to what occurred in Amsterdam? Why do almost none of them know about this early breakthrough? One reason may be the sequel. Some Dutch AIDS activists had all along expressed qualms about promoting "absti-nence," but after 1991 the message changed. Now it said that con-doms reduced risk just as well as no anal sex at all, a claim of utter irresponsibility.[7] I knew that because I would soon be working in the condom world myself.

Adventures in the Skin Coverage Trade

Unlike the ever-sensible Dutch, the U.S. government responded slowly to AIDS, as if it were a pest that might depart if we ignored it. Some people opposed *any* response, saying gays had brought the disease on themselves and deserved it. In 1987 the government finally began to move internationally, launching two global preven-tion programs: AIDSCOM, for "behavior change," and AIDSTECH for operational research, blood safety, and testing methods.

The firm that sent me to Swaziland, the Academy for Educational Development, carried out AIDSCOM. Its first director was an HIV-positive gay activist from South Africa who died a few years into the program. In general, the early AIDS professionals came from the ranks of gay activists—usually with little overseas experience—and from the family-planning world. These people, like myself, had plenty of overseas experience but none in AIDS. I was friends with one of the original AIDSCOM teams; indeed, I worked as an AIDS-COM consultant for a while in the early 1990s. My gay colleague was convinced that a lot of male gay sex was going on in Africa; it was just hidden because of the intense stigma against homosexuality in Africa and the Third World generally. Early safe-sex ambassadors like him felt it was important to prove that gay men were a significant population in Africa. The Academy for Educational Development published a book listing this as a major achievement for America's first global AIDS prevention effort.

Between 1986 and 1989, I worked in condom marketing, for John Short and Associates and then for The Futures Group, the second largest contraceptive social marketing company. "Social marketing" meant marketing with a socially beneficial goal. The idea was, if products that are *bad* for people's health (like Coca-Cola) are available in every cranny of the planet, from Tibet to Easter Island, why not use the same forces to bring them products that are *good* for them (like vitamins and oral rehydration salts)? This approach rests on the fact that free-market forces such as the law of supply and demand have proven far more efficient than government distribution systems. However, a key part of this equation received insufficient attention: demand. There is clear demand for coke (the cola or the narcotic), but demand drops off steeply with condoms and oral rehydration salts. Still, we tried to reach as many people as possible and thus promoted birth control with low, subsidized prices through well-established wholesale and retail channels, in both formal and informal sectors.

When AIDS arrived, we had our first prevention idea right at hand—the condom! As AIDS spread worldwide, we envisioned exponential growth in sales. And we could market the condom as "dual purpose," meaning it would prevent both pregnancy and HIV infection. Two for the price of one. As it happened, though, this AIDS prevention idea was also the *last* many people would have.

By 1985, USAID had become so interested in social marketing that it launched a twenty-one-million-dollar global program to promote contraceptives for birth control: Social Marketing for Change (SOMARC). As the AIDS pandemic evolved, agencies relied more and more on social marketing and similar approaches to spread condom use as widely as possible. The technique went mainstream, and such market research methods as focus groups became standard in public health and even anthropology.

I was the token anthropologist on the SOMARC Advisory Board, before I went to work full time on the actual project. In my advisory role I argued that Africa was another world and that we needed to understand sexual behaviors, gender relations, and fertility beliefs on several levels—from the individual to the peer group to family, lineage, clan, and to the broader society and culture. But social marketing was new and glitzy then, and it brought Madison Avenue pros together with family-planning experts. The ad guys believed they had market-research techniques that could quickly reveal the consumer habits ("psychographics" was a favorite buzzword) of segmented target audiences, typically stratified by socioeconomic factors. They had developed the formula in the West, but felt it would apply to Africans and Asians just as well.

Few people in anthropology and any other relevant fields critically examined the premises of the AIDS prevention model then developing. The model focused on condoms and their marketing rather than on understanding sexual behavior and ways to influence it. Indeed, everyone seemed to assume that sexual behavior change was simply outside the discussion, too difficult to achieve or just beyond tampering with. I mean, what was our Sexual Revolution for? I knew that the real challenge would lie in getting everyone to use condoms consistently. No one had ever succeeded at it in general populations as distinct from special risk groups. Even if it were possible, somehow, we all knew condoms were not especially effective. That's why we had generally promoted other birth-control methods. So essentially we were setting sail across the sea in a vessel that had never gotten far from shore.

Nonetheless, the safe-sex message (later changed to "safer-sex" in a nod to the facts) became: as long as you use a condom (especially one provided by us, so you can be sure of quality), you can keep enjoying all the sex you want. A poster photographed by a colleague in Guinea as late as 2006 showed pictographically that penis + vagina + condom = "no risk" of disease. It also showed penis + rectum + condom = "no risk." This of course is ludicrous and highly dangerous (I'll speak more on this point later). And soon, through a series of steps, I found myself more or less in charge of the contraceptive social marketing program in the Dominican Republic. I made quite a name for myself there.

In 1987, I became head of a condom market study in the DR. My company had used social marketing very successfully to promote the Pill, and I developed innovative research methods to prove we were reaching our target audience in the Dominican Republic: the lower-middle class. I published some of the first peer-reviewed papers on the DR program, indeed, on any SOMARC program. The DR was ahead of the rest of the world in dealing with AIDS. In 1986 and 1987 it rolled out a bold, insightful program that included handing out brochures to tourists as they arrived, warning that AIDS was circulating in the country and they should avoid prostitutes. For those visitors who scorned this advice, the mass media aired blunt condom ads, and every hotel and motel had two free condoms next to the Gideon Bible. I even discovered that AIDS campaign folks from the DR's Ministry of Health had met privately with top Catholic Church authorities and reached an understanding that the Church would not openly oppose condom promotion because latex could prevent this fatal, incurable STD (or so we thought).

In February 1988, I presented a paper on my DR findings at the American Association for the Advancement of Science (AAAS) annual conference in Boston. By then I'd learned that one can go publicity fishing. To divine what the press wants to hear, you simply imagine various possible headlines. I mentioned in my paper that when one compared our survey findings with those from a similar random sample study of American men, lo and behold, lower-middle class Dominican men knew more about AIDS and how to prevent it than American men did! The DR had also doubled condom prevalence rates in a single year (although it went from low to not-so-low, as a *Washington Post* reporter had me clarify).

But remember, it was early 1988 and all the news about AIDS so far had been bad, outside the barely noticed Dutch study. My paper might have been the first promising report the world had heard. And AIDS World picked up exactly the message it had been pining for: if we were willful and energetic enough, we could swiftly spread condom use and beat back the pestilence. There was hope!

I was pulled into a press conference and interviewed by National Public Radio about my extraordinary findings. The AAAS sent word out on its clipping service, and over the next several weeks scores of laudatory articles about Ted Green's research appeared in newspapers around the United States, Latin America, and Europe. Front-page articles came out in the major Dominican Republic dailies, raining praise on the gringo "doctor" who had put the DR in the AIDS prevention vanguard. The *Journal of the American Medical Association* wrote a favorable piece about me, and I got a raise and a promotion. I was the bright new star of an industry just then coalescing around AIDS prevention.

This time, I really *was* ready to tackle the world. But I would fall so far from my early poster-boy status that I'd be seen as a traitor to the Condom Code.

The change actually began later that same year, in 1988. I was invited to contribute an article to one of the first books on the social and policy dimensions of AIDS in Africa. Many other anthropologists also wrote pieces for this volume, including Tom Barton, Francis Conant, Charles Good, Ann Gowan, Edward Greeley, Priscilla Reining, and Brooke Schoepf. Some of us urged more research on the growing African plague, which we realized was a mosaic of diverse epidemics. Relying on my knowledge of Africa, condoms, and AIDS, I wrote: "Regarding necessary changes in behavior: (1) Both unmarried and married men will have to become monogamous or severely restrict their number of sexual partners. Women will have to be empowered to refuse sexual intercourse to a far greater extent than they are at present."[8] I also mentioned a need for condoms, and I said we had to mobilize a cross-section of groups in society, including both faith-based organizations and family-planning associations. There was nothing arcane about these ideas. Sleep with fewer people and you cut your chance of exposure to a virus spread by intercourse. Avoid sex with suspect partners and you do the same. Mobilize more groups and a campaign grows more effective.

But almost no one listened.

Twelve years later, in February 2000, my Swazi friend Joe and I were walking down the main street in Mbabane, Swaziland. We came across a pal of his, a fellow journalist named Knowledge (his real name). Knowledge put his hands on Joe's neck and asked, "How are your glands? Is that stuff helping?"

Joe looked embarrassed and mumbled, "Sure, fine," and kept walking. I asked Joe if he was sick. He said it was just a little minor something, it was under control, and he quickly changed the subject.

I never saw him again. Joe died of AIDS around Christmas of that year. I was living in Washington then, and he never wrote or phoned to tell me he had AIDS or even that he was seriously ill. If he had, I would have found a way to get him antiretroviral drugs, as he must have known, and he would still be alive today. Such is the magnitude of shame and stigma associated with AIDS in most of southern Africa, even today. Swaziland has the highest HIV infection rate in the world. Sam's friend Knowledge died of AIDS in 2001.

They might both be alive if they had lived in Uganda.

PART II

UGANDA

We are being told that only a thin piece of rubber stands between us and the death of our continent. I feel that condoms have a role to play as a means of protection, especially in couples who are HIV-positive, but they cannot become the main means of stemming the tide of AIDS.

YOWERI MUSEVENI
president of Uganda, 1991

CHAPTER 3

The Twenty-five-cent Solution

I first visited Uganda in March 1993. I had been collaborating with the Tanzanian psychiatrist Dr. Lucy Nkya and a contractor from the United States Agency for International Development (USAID), (now Dr.) Anne Outwater, on a study of sex workers in Morogoro, a town inland from the coast of Tanzania. People here and in many parts of Africa initially blamed AIDS on witchcraft, but by 1993 most realized it was a sexually transmitted disease. The scholarly literature on prostitution in this country was scant. We did a survey in a slum compound with some two hundred sex workers who offered short-time sex for about forty U.S. cents a tumble, mostly to itinerant truck drivers—the very subpopulation that had spread HIV all over the continent.

Our program protocols called for testing the sex workers for STDs, including HIV. We found that most of these sex workers were HIV-infected, and in fact most of them would die over the next few years. Dr. Nkya had fought successfully against the prevailing practice of refusing to bury prostitutes in Christian cemeteries. It was because of their love of Dr. Lucy that the sex workers consented to be interviewed—and they poured out their lives to the interviewers. I actually picked up a bad case of scabies from shaking hands with grateful prostitutes and holding their babies, but I later managed to get their stories published in six installments, as pure narratives without the interruption of analysis or interpretation.[1]

When I finished the first phase of the Tanzanian work, I went to Uganda for a week on a side consulting assignment. Uganda is a landlocked nation with fabled lakes. To its south is isle-studded Lake Victoria, an inland sea full of crocodiles, pirates, sea flies, and parasitic worms. The Nile originates here, flowing north across the great Sahara, past the Pyramids, and into the Mediterranean. To the west rise the glacial Ruwenzori peaks, also called the Mountains of the Moon; legendary in ancient times, they are one of the last places on earth to see gorillas. Southern Uganda is lush and flat, rich with palms, rice paddies, and banana trees, and the capital, Kampala, is a hilly city with streets shaded by trees where storks nest. It's a beautiful land.

But it had suffered decades of brutality and chaos. Ruthless kleptocrats like Milton Obote and the murderous Idi Amin had soaked the country in blood and destroyed almost everything that worked. Yoweri Museveni overthrew Obote in 1986, and he had brought stability and sense to the top position. Of course, he too is an autocrat, and it's probably not good he's still there after a quarter century, but considering the kind of leadership Uganda and too many other African countries have suffered, I for one am not complaining too loudly.

Museveni at once faced a new enemy: AIDS. To our knowledge, it first appeared in Uganda in 1982, among fishermen and merchants in the Rakai district east of Lake Victoria. By 1985 the disease had spread widely, and before long most Ugandans knew people who had died of "Slim," as they called it (because victims wasted away). In 1988, Uganda had the highest percentage of HIV infections on earth. It reached 30 percent among women receiving prenatal care in some major cities—a staggering rate for a then-100 percent lethal disease that a mother could also give to her babies. By 1991, 21 percent of urban Ugandans (or 15 percent overall, once we factor in the lower rates in rural areas) were HIV infected.

Yet my Ugandan informants told me they felt they were beating back the disease. White folks raised their brows at such claims, but today we know the Ugandans were correct: *incidence* (that is, the rate of new infections) seems to have peaked around 1988 and 1989, and *prevalence* (the overall percentage of the population infected) in 1992. Incidence usually falls first because it can drop while the prevalence grows. Imagine a hose pouring water into a pool. If you reduce the inflow (the incidence), the water level in the pool (the prevalence) will keep rising anyway until more is going out (the deaths). To fall, the pool must lose more water than it gets. So prevalence sums up a whole history, but incidence shows us the critical, immediate HIV trends. Incidence is even more important today, when antiretroviral therapy (ART) is keeping infected persons alive much longer. ART normally increases prevalence, because fewer people are dying, but incidence can still be either rising or falling. Unfortunately, researchers collect data much more routinely on prevalence than incidence.

In Uganda foreign AIDS experts doubted any decline was occurring because they knew how few condoms were circulating in 1993. Condom social marketing was not yet functioning as a national program, and few condoms were available outside of Kampala. Social Marketing for Change (SOMARC) ran Uganda's first condom social marketing, and I knew its strategies well and had full access to its data. Something other than condoms had to be saving lives.

As an anthropologist, I did commonsense things most technical experts don't bother with or have confidence in. For example, I went around and spoke to nurses and doctors at sexually transmitted disease (STD) clinics, health and education officials, traditional healers, birth attendants, anyone who might spot trends, and basically asked, "What's going on?" I heard—and saw—that Uganda in 1993 had created a novel type of prevention program. The nation was promoting fidelity and delay of "sexual debut" (a rare case of jargon more charming than the common phrase: "loss of virginity"). I could sense the excitement among Ugandans that these efforts were paying off. Fewer adults were going to bars, having casual sex, and having multiple partners, and more young people were postponing sex. As behavior changed, fewer men with STDs were presenting at clinics. My Ugandan informants told me that people had become very afraid of getting AIDS.

Meanwhile, most of the rest of Africa was pretending that AIDS was not a threat. In former Zaire, the French acronym for AIDS, SIDA, was said to stand for "Syndrome Imaginaire pour Décourager les Amoureux" ("Imaginary Syndrome to Discourage Lovers"). Neighboring Uganda had to take deliberate steps to cut through the denial that Ugandans were at risk of this new disease. It was seen by many as an American gay disease (not that many Africans knew what "gay" meant)—or at least an American plot to spoil fun, force condom use, and thereby deplete the population of black people.

This could be the story of the century, I thought. So I wrote a memo to the USAID office (or "mission") in Kampala, saying that the Ugandan government was emphasizing two interventions that *we* were not supporting: fidelity and delay. Because they seemed to be working, I suggested that we start backing these interventions. In my 1993 consultant report to USAID, I wrote: "There is anecdotal evidence that STD incidence has significantly decreased in Uganda in the last year or two. While this may reflect wishful or politically motivated thinking, it would be extremely significant if this were true. If a high AIDS-prevalence country like Uganda shows a significant decline in STDs (presumably a harbinger of a later decline in HIV seroprevalence) *in the absence of a male condom prevalence rate of over 5 percent,* it might suggest that *other* types of behavior change ('premarital chastity,' 'zero grazing,' marital fidelity, abstinence, nonpenetrative and other safer sexual practices) can significantly affect STD incidence if not HIV incidence."[2]

I got no response. In retrospect, this marks the beginning of my alienation from USAID, my career lifeblood for many years before 2001, when my antiestablishment AIDS activism became a full-time campaign.

I made a second trip to Uganda in 1996, to evaluate a family-planning project focused on condom distribution. I noticed that the foreign AIDS prevention effort still seemed pretty clueless about the factors that made Uganda's approach special. It was pushing the same old interventions as if we were in San Francisco or New York. And two years later, in 1998, I saw some data in a World Bank book on global AIDS, coedited by health economist Mead Over, that showed an unexpected association between education and wealth and higher infection rates. That is, richer, better-schooled Africans got HIV more often, a pattern seen as early as 1983. The same chapter noted an association between condom use and greater levels of education and wealth. The more advantaged also used condoms more often.[3]

I was riveted. The document did not go further and say, "The better educated and wealthier are more apt to use condoms *and* get HIV." I remember thinking, *I understand. No one wants to admit that our main strategy, condoms, might actually be backfiring.* In a sidebar the authors sketched a bleak future for Africa—one of doom, defeat, despair, and death. We seemed powerless to make even a dent in AIDS. Yet there might be one emerging success story: Uganda. There was an urgent need for someone to go to Uganda, to look carefully at HIV trends and behavioral data, and to search for links between interventions and behavioral trends.

"Wow, I'd sure like to be the one who gets to do that!" I enthused to my wife. "But I don't have any connections at the Bank. It's not the same universe as USAID."

A few months later the phone rang. It was a contractor asking if I was available for a World Bank assignment overseas, in November and December of 1998. I turned him down because I didn't want to spend a whole month abroad just then. The caller said he quite understood and was about to hang up when I added, "By the way, what is the assignment?" It was of course the Dream Job for the guy who thought he knew the secret of Uganda's success.

I wound up spending a full month in Uganda, where I dug up and examined all available evidence, from the epidemiological to behavioral, looking for preliminary links between behavior change and interventions that promoted it. I saw convincing evidence of *primary* behavior change: just as Ugandans had told me earlier, people were having fewer sex partners, and young people were delaying sexual debut. In fact, according to the World Health Organization (WHO) and UNAIDS (United Nations AIDS, easily confused with the much wealthier USAID), from 1989 to 1995 the percentage of Ugandan women with at least one casual partner dropped from 16 percent to 6 percent. Among Ugandan men it fell from 35 percent to 15 percent. Strikingly, the men reporting three or more partners declined from 15 percent in 1989 to 3 percent in 1995.

But don't people lie in sex surveys? Some do, but we have to start with our best empirical evidence and then triangulate it with other findings, such as medical evidence. And these findings, as well as the less tangible general perception, also supported the decrease. This change was coming cheap. At least in the early stage, it cost $21,676,000 over five years, or twenty-five cents per person, per year.[4] Meanwhile, we in the West were pouring hundreds of millions (soon, billions) of dollars into expensive interventions that seemed to have no effect, and still don't, some thirty years into the pandemic.

When I finished in Uganda, I wrote my report. I knew that one of the many things the AIDS establishment would not like about my findings was that "we," the major donors, had not been promoting the behavior change that was occurring. I sensed there might be some political or ideological resistance to my findings, but because the epidemic was ghastly and most people in AIDS work mean well, I didn't worry too much about it.

I needed a clear, simple moniker to capture the difference between Uganda's program and business-as-usual AIDS preven-tion. Around 1985 or 1986 a rather obscure health educator in Ohio named Steven Sroka had coined the abbreviation ABC—abstain, be faithful, or use a condom—to help introduce AIDS prevention in local schools. WHO and other international organizations learned of the term and sometimes used it to mollify conservative Third

World leaders who complained that "AIDS prevention" really meant handing out condoms to kids. "No, no," Western donors could say, "we promote A and B and only then, C-for-condoms!"

I believe I was the first person to call Uganda's program "ABC." The name stuck and then became official U.S. policy (ironically, before Ugandan). In 1998, I naively thought that including C-for-condoms would keep powerful interests from dismissing the A and B parts, allow the West to save face and condom sales to continue. Of course, if anyone had read my memo in 1993, the major donors could by 1998 have been taking credit for Africa's first clear success story.

In this 1998 report to the World Bank, my first four recommendations focused on fidelity. I wrote them in clear English and no one could mistake their import. Again, I heard nothing. I soon found out that two former WHO epidemiologists later working for Cambridge University, Rand Stoneburner and Daniel Low-Beer, had reached conclusions similar to my own. I would not meet them for another two years, but when I did, we had similar stories to compare. They too had thought that the world would welcome their findings. How could the world *not?* After all, our evidence showed we could prevent AIDS in Africa far more cheaply and successfully than anyone had dared imagine. We could stop the holocaust. These guys felt we were witnessing one the greatest violations of human rights of the century: we knew how to prevent AIDS and yet we weren't taking action.

It would take Stoneburner and Low-Beer six years to find a major journal (*Science*) willing to publish their findings. They were also summarily fired from South Africa's largest AIDS program after their careful, objective evaluation found that the program not only was failing, but that it also seemed to be associated with *increased* teen sex and HIV infection. It's not as if they threatened to go public with these results, but the Kaiser Foundation seized their computers and impounded their evaluation report in the hard drives. Then the foundation went to the new Global Fund to ask for, and get, some sixty million dollars to run its "successful" program for another five years.

There may be some justice in the world, however. Five years after *that*, directors of the same project went back to the Global Fund. By then, Low-Beer was a key official in funding decisions. He showed project directors their own stated objectives and asked innocently, "Have you achieved a single one of these?" The result: no more funds.

Stoneburner would later estimate that the ABC program might have saved 3.2 million lives in South Africa from 2000 to 2010 and prevented 80 percent of HIV infections in the worst-hit lands of the sub-Sahara.[5] What was Uganda's secret?

Prevention by Full Court Press

Uganda began its program in 1986, after Fidel Castro placed a phone call to President Museveni. Some sixty Ugandan soldiers had trained in Cuba and the health authorities had tested them. A high percentage, Castro told the new president, had HIV antibodies. This news greatly disturbed Museveni and he set to work at once. Milton Obote had recently fled the country, and the world still deemed Uganda a ghoulish outcast. It received little money from the West and had few Western public-health experts on hand. So Museveni launched his own program.

I met with Museveni in September 2004 and had a chance to ask him some details about how and why prevalence declined dramatically.

He is an imposing, gracious, intelligent man, and he was Africa's (and probably the world's) first AIDS activist who was also a head of state. Here is the recipe that could have saved so many lives:

- Extensive public promotion of fidelity and delay of sexual debut (that is, behavior change)
- Bold leadership at the highest level
- Community participation, with open, face-to-face discussions about AIDS
- Involvement of religious leaders

- Involvement of people living with HIV
- Deliberate use of "fear appeals" to spur behavior change
- Fight against AIDS-associated stigma
- AIDS education in primary schools, to reach children before they become sexually active
- Special targeting of women and youth

These tenets may sound pretty mundane. As H. L. Mencken once said: "The problem with the truth is that it is mainly uncomfortable and often dull." Yet put together, these preventive ideas were magic.

President Museveni created the thirty-person National Committee for the Prevention of AIDS in 1986, and the AIDS Control Program (ACP) began in 1987. The ACP developed a training structure (including trainers of trainers) to inform groups throughout society. It also began printing huge numbers of training manuals, pamphlets, posters, and other educational materials. The next major organization was the Uganda AIDS Commission (UAC), launched in 1991 and 1992. Both it and the ACP focused on the local community. They stressed that AIDS prevention was the responsibility of neighbor support systems, schools, religious associations, professional groups, family networks, and community groups. The government and a few large organizations alone couldn't stop the disease.

The Messengers

Messenger #1 was Museveni himself. From the outset he began mentioning AIDS at every opportunity. So did his wife and key advisers. Indeed, civil servants (and Africa always employs too many) were told they had to talk about AIDS every time they spoke in public. It became everyone's patriotic duty to defeat this new enemy, this "snake that crawled into our house" and "lion that entered our village." Uganda is a highly religious country, and its citizens simply did not talk about sex freely or in mixed company, so this approach was critical to make discussion acceptable and spread information. If

Museveni and the people in government were speaking freely about it, others could too, without standing out. Most world leaders at the time, including Ronald Reagan, and a bit later, Nelson Mandela, were silent about AIDS while they were in office.

The faith-based organizations (FBOs) were among the first and most prominent NGOs working in African AIDS. When it came to prevention strategies, they clearly preferred fidelity and delay, yet because foreign donors firmly believed these approaches were ineffective, they sidelined these potentially powerful partners. In Uganda most people belonged to the Roman Catholic Church or the Anglican Church (the Church of Uganda), followed by the Islamic *umma* ("community of Islam"). Relatively few independent churches or sects existed. So when the three faith communities developed programs together to encourage behavior change, they could reach the great majority of Ugandans. USAID in Uganda was willing to fund prevention programs run by Anglicans and Muslims, but not Catholics, because of a predictable impasse over condoms. Yet by funding any FBOs, USAID/Uganda was ahead of their counterparts in other countries. At the local level efforts varied, but in many communities pastors or imams spoke about AIDS and faithfulness, both in their regular services and sometimes during or after funerals for people who had died of AIDS.

Museveni was clear on this matter. He said, "We need everyone"— all resources available—to fight the terrible scourge of AIDS. In the nongovernmental sector, FBOs are the major players. We *must* involve them. Yes, the FBOs might cite scripture and talk about right and wrong when promoting abstinence and fidelity. They would make value judgments. But this strategy worked, and even more, it did not stigmatize the ill, as many feared it would. Uganda found itself ahead of other African countries in destigmatizing AIDS. Uganda bombarded citizens with the message from all sides. It used every communication channel available—electronic, print, interpersonal—because each had strengths and drawbacks. Fighting along a broad front, the government knew, yielded maximum exposure and synergy, especially if it used the channels in complementary and mutually reinforcing ways. Research has shown that multiple channels yield an effect greater than the sum of parts. One plus one exceeds two.

The media focused intensely on AIDS, and the TV, radio, and print coverage was thorough. But delivery went even further. Posters and billboards appeared, and citizens saw plays and music performances about AIDS. Competitions took place with prizes for the best poems, songs, or plays about AIDS. The government spread the message in several Ugandan languages, to reach everyone. This campaign penetrated deep into Ugandan society. It pervaded every sector and almost every public organization—such as district health teams, schools, local councils, youth organizations, women's groups, NGOs, and prisons. In 1988 the popular Ugandan singer Philly Lutaaya revealed he had AIDS, and he spent his last haggard days bravely touring the country to speak out for fidelity. People saw him wasting away before their eyes. Philly would say, "You people don't have to end up like me. You can save yourselves."

Traditional healers took part as well. Although they were happy to be asked to openly join in preventing AIDS, most African governments have policies of benign neglect with regard to healers. However, the Museveni regime developed a model program of collaboration. As it happens, one of the herbal medicines the healers developed for (AIDS-related) herpes was found through a clinical trial to be as effective as the leading, expensive antiviral drug for the illness. The results were published in a peer-reviewed journal.[6]

Other countries have followed versions of this multipronged strategy. But as comparative Demographic and Health Survey (DHS, the gold standard) analysis shows, Uganda stands out among African nations because: (1) it emphasized primary behavior change, and (2) it stressed and achieved a high level of interpersonal (or face-to-face), community-based, culturally tailored communication about AIDS and how to best prevent it.[7] This approach also succeeded because Africans place more value on collective responsibility—that is, the family, lineage, and clan—than on individual rights, especially the right to engage in socially disapproved behaviors. A proverb among Nguni-speaking groups of southern Africa says: *Umuntu ngumuntu ngabantu* ("A person is a person because of other people"). It's John Donne's "No man is an island," but more emphatically. Others—our friends, neighbors, living lineage members, and ancestors—therefore create our humanity.

The Message: Be Careful and Be Afraid

In Uganda the message was clear: "Be faithful," "Love carefully," and "Practice zero grazing"—the last a reference to tethering a bull in its own paddock. If you are in a relationship, honor it. Don't stray. If you are single, wait till marriage for sex or have only one partner. If you do have sex outside a relationship, always use a condom. Nearly everywhere else, the condom message came first and probably nothing else came with it, except in later years we added "get tested" and "get your STD diagnosed and treated." We spread this use-a-condom message everywhere, to all audiences, no matter the culture.

A 1991 external USAID evaluation of the AIDS Control Program found that Ugandans remembered "Love faithfully"—aimed largely at men—more often than "Stick to one partner," "Zero grazing," "Love carefully," or any other slogan. The messages went beyond catchphrases. Groups gave people accurate information about AIDS and how they might get it. Through newspaper or radio stories, posters, pamphlets, fables, skits, and other means, they emphasized people's susceptibility to AIDS if they did not love carefully. They highlighted the consequences, the long feebleness leading to death, but also the terrible orphaning of children, the loss of skilled workers and entrepreneurs for the economy, and the cratering impact on society. These messages were straightforward: one need only contrast the simple fidelity-and-abstinence poster from the Uganda Ministry of Education with the snazzy, American-created comic book in the superhero genre, featuring Captain Condom and Lady Latex defeating a gang of diseased bad guys. Uganda dealt directly with risky behavior, rather than dancing around it or ignoring it. It also relied on its own common sense, resources, and intimate knowledge of its own culture; Westerners used Western-created media, concepts, and themes, no doubt with Western epidemics in mind.

Uganda also used outright scare tactics. Officials repeated slogans like "Have sex and die." They posted billboards all over the nation showing coffins, skulls, and crossbones. At every public meeting, Museveni said, "I would shout at them, 'You are going to die if you don't stop this [having multiple sexual partners]. You are going to die!'" Dr. Sam Okware, the first director of the ACP, explained: "We drove fear into people." The idea was to vaporize denial about AIDS. The emphasis was on fear of *getting* AIDS—not fear of the person with HIV. Citizens had to treat the infected with kindness and compassion because, in the words of a popular Philly Lutaaya song, "Today it's me. Tomorrow it might be you." In focus groups people often mentioned a drum that beat somberly on the radio many times per day, signaling the reading of names of individuals who had died that day. The country was in crisis, the message said. Even fifteen years later people quickly recalled its beat, and its visceral impact on them.[8]

It may seem hard to believe, but among Western AIDS experts it is almost an article of faith that fear appeals flop, and even boomerang, a la *Reefer Madness*. Indeed, AIDS workers mocked fear appeals as "amateurish," "misguided," and even immoral. It was clear that on a basic level they didn't believe their own arguments. Indeed, they regularly used fear appeals themselves (even to convince others that fear appeals wouldn't work). Consider this response from the manager of the World Bank's AIDS Portfolio in Africa to yet another "expert" report on African AIDS: "It should be called 'The Day the Moon-size Meteor Strikes Earth.' Not a single new word or shred of data, not a single insight, nor a constructive suggestion. Just rehashed, undifferentiated fear-mongering."[9] And he was not unusual in rejecting this message.

Kim Witte, a well-known authority on fear appeals at Michigan State University, conducted a meta-analysis of research on fear arousal and hard-to-change behaviors. She and her colleagues found that fear arousal, if linked with self-efficacy—that is, knowing clear and doable ways to avoid the threat—can indeed motivate behavior change. If I say, "Wall Street is collapsing and a global recession is coming," you probably won't try to stop it, because nothing you can do will work. But if I say, "A rabid dog is coming down the block. Stay inside," you can do that. Yet another meta-analysis of thirty-five published studies on a wide range of topics, subjects, and communications vehicles concluded that "increases in fear are consistently associated with increases in acceptance [of the recommended action]."[10]

Kim and I eventually published an article that brought together Uganda's experience and the literature on fear appeals, although it was rejected time after time in the review process. Many reviewers expressed offense at an article that challenged so many accepted beliefs. We only managed to squeak through peer review in a non-AIDS journal, and probably because my coauthor was on the journal's advisory board.[11] Even then, I was asked to meet the editor for lunch, and I may have passed some sort of test (yes, Ted Green is not a conservative). Understand: I have published many articles in my career. Personal interviews aren't typically part of the process.

Focus on the Vulnerable

Uganda's program singled out two audiences in particular: young people and women. As early as 1987, its schools began stressing the danger of AIDS along with self-efficacy, the means to avoid it. Indeed, the government required all schools to teach AIDS prevention, and the key message for youth was: delay sex. Museveni told them not to rush into contaminating contact. They had their whole lives ahead, and only a fool risked early death for sex. In addition, schools involved youth in activities like dramas and songs, and encouraged students to take information home to parents.

Museveni also addressed the "sugar daddy" phenomenon common in Africa, whereby older men take very young women as mistresses and give them benefits in return. The Ugandan government made sex with a minor under eighteen a criminal offense and gave sex with very young girls an excellent, stigmatizing name: "defilement." How successful was this effort? HIV prevalence declined more among people between fifteen and nineteen than in any other age group. A study of city youth found a two-year delay in sexual debut among people fifteen to twenty-four.[12] (A recent randomized, controlled study in the United States also found evidence that such a strategy can work.[13]) One reason seems to be that abstinence is a much easier sell to people uninitiated in sex.

A sea change occurred even among more experienced students. According to field researchers' stories, young male Ugandans who once deemed an STD a badge of manhood now saw it as a sign of stupidity. John Kiwanuka is today a New York public-health physician responsible for HIV/AIDS policy at the Africa-America Institute, but in 1986 he was a medical student at Kampala's Makerere University. "My friends and I wanted to party and celebrate. We had girlfriends," he said. Then the fidelity campaign began. "There was a dramatic change among students in 1987 and 1988," he noted. "I took precautions. My friends changed their behavior. The ones that didn't, succumbed to the disease."[14] This new caution was extremely important, because the period between sexual debut and marriage (or an equivalent commitment) is the time of greatest risk.

The program also targeted women and took steps to improve their status in a number of ways, such as enforcing rape and defilement laws, providing special rules to get more women into higher education, urging them to organize associations and then working with them, and telling men to respect and be true to their wives. The ABC program encouraged women to demand fidelity and to leave their husbands if they betrayed them. Sophia Mukasa Monico, a Ugandan and now a UNAIDS representative for Swaziland, observed that the all-out initiative changed Ugandan women, made them take more responsibility for their own lives. "Wives told their husbands to be faithful, use a condom, even in marriage, or there would be no sex," she said. "Many women in Uganda had celibate marriages or moved out on their own."[15] By as early as 1987, in fact, some women were saying that the anti-HIV program had saved their marriages. In the Kampala suburb of Bugolobi a young mother of three stated: "There has been a positive change in our marriage. My husband stays at home much more. And I encourage him to do so by enthusiastically keeping him informed of the latest gossip about Slim victims."[16] Other articles observed that AIDS had crashed the market for prostitutes and that fewer men sought to lure barmaids into brief relationships.

The DHS asks a question to women all over the developing world: "Do you feel you are justified in refusing to have sex with your husband because . . . (for reasons ranging from knowing the husband has an STD to just not being in the mood)." A greater percentage of women in Uganda answer yes to these questions than anywhere else in Africa. This program sounds highly feminist, yet a colleague of mine struggled to get a coauthored feminist perspective on ABC accepted in a peer-reviewed journal. In the end the free online Public Library of Science (PLoS) published the article, but it circulated mostly in a summary form, which actually twisted their findings so they seemed to support condoms. Indeed, one of many arguments used to attack Uganda's ABC program was that "it does not apply to women." Another argument was the greater absurdity that it is harmful for women.

And the misunderstanding ran even deeper, and still does.

CHAPTER 4

The Crossroads
and the Cul-de-sac

AIDS in Africa has bewildered the West for decades. It seems to act like a different disease there, striking a new array of victims and spreading far beyond its silos in the West. From the outset people have wondered, Why is African AIDS mainly heterosexual? And why are the infection rates so astronomical in some parts? The answer is subtle and still eludes many: it's all about networks. To most people's surprise, HIV is actually hard to transmit—much, much harder than, say, gonorrhea and other common STDs. For heterosexuals the risk per act of intercourse is around one in a thousand, or even less. Infection thus usually requires a great many acts—and a person is far more likely to get HIV from an ongoing partner than from a prostitute, if both have it. Hence multiple concurrent partners, such as married sugar daddies with mistresses, raise the risk. More risk from one's regular partner than from a prostitute? This goes against our gut instinct, centuries of thought, and even biblical wisdom. But if multiple, concurrent partnerships are common, sexual networks can take shape.

Consider this pattern: Suppose Alice is sleeping regularly with Ben and Charles, Ben with Diane and Ellen, and Charles with Frieda, Gloria, and Helen. And suppose Diane, Ellen, Frieda, Gloria, and Helen are each sleeping with two or more people themselves. A web arises. Each person is like a fork or crossroads, and the virus becomes like a car on an interstate. It can go anywhere. Outside of sub-Saharan

Africa sexually active people are generally monogamous, although they change partners, some fairly often. Thus, although Americans and Europeans average more sex partners over their lifetimes than Africans, they usually have them one at a time—that is, Ann begins and ends a relationship with Bob, then begins and ends one with Charles, and so forth. We call this pattern "serial monogamy." The HIV rate in the United States has never reached 1 percent.

In contrast, a fairly substantial minority of Africans, even when married, have one and sometimes two or more lovers on the side. For instance, men often migrate from nations like Swaziland and Botswana to work in the cities and mines of South Africa. It's a magnet for labor, because it is the only industrialized country on the continent. Many of these migrants interrupt their marriages and leave their wives in the village for months or years at a time. A significant minority of men and women establish a second ongoing relationship—the man with somebody where he's working, and the woman eventually with another man in the village who helps pay school fees for the children.

In Botswana, for example, 43 percent of young men and 17 percent of women in one survey reported they currently had two or more regular lovers. A recent study in Malawi found that 65 percent of sexually active people in seven villages on Likoma Island were linked into one giant sexual web, even though the average number of concurrent partners was three.[1] Only 20 percent of couples were mutually monogamous. In such a widespread, near-invisible network, one person's health affects almost everyone else's. The Likoma percentage is unusually high, but it's no coincidence that AIDS has flared so out of control in these areas.

The High-risk Window

Networks are hazardous for another reason as well. The transmissibility rate of one in a thousand is an oft-cited average that obscures some rather extreme variations, because a variety of factors affect the chance of passing on the virus. One factor is male circumcision. Other factors include:

- Viral load of the HIV-positive partner
- Presence of another STD, especially one causing open sores
- Site of intercourse (anal is much riskier than vaginal)
- Practice of "dry sex," with vaginal drying agents
- Time of intercourse—that is, whether it occurs during menstruation
- Presence or absence of coercion
- Correct use or nonuse of a condom

Viral load seems the most important of these factors in Africa. Viral load is the measurable amount of virus in a bodily fluid such as blood or semen. It rises and falls in a predictable course. When HIV enters the body, it bushwhacks the immune system. Lacking effective enemies, the HIV population explodes over the next several weeks to months, as rabbits once did in Australia. The newly infected person becomes highly contagious, yet the victim shows few signs of illness. He or she does not feel sick, and standard HIV tests will not flag the ailment, because the immune system has not yet churned out the antibodies they measure. So the risk of infection per act of heterosexual intercourse is far greater—roughly 1 in 10 to 1 in 125—if one has the bad luck to encounter a partner in the window just after infection. According to some researchers, up to half of all transmissions occur during this phase, depending on the type of epidemic and the nature of sexual relationships.[2]

When the immune system finally starts pumping out antibodies, they drive HIV levels down for the next five or more years. Infectiousness drops and a long race to exhaustion ensues between HIV and the immune cells (today with the help of antiretrovirals). When HIV begins to prevail, the body seems to lose its ability to forge more antibodies. We then become helpless before even small-time infections that normally pose little threat to us, like flus or gastroenteritis. Viral load soars again, but this time the person is visibly ill. He or she may also have less sex, either because of lower drive or the wariness of potential partners who see the ravages of disease. Hence the final stage may account for relatively few transmissions. But the initial open window lets the virus race through sexual networks. So Alice quickly infects Ben, who infects Diane, and so on. A hyperepidemic can occur. In lands with serial monogamy, however, the bug gets trapped in relationship capsules for months or even years at a time. The victim does put all future sex partners at risk, but the threat is less, because the acute stage has usually passed.

The Snippers Effect

I first argued in 1988 that number of sexual partners was the key factor in populationwide epidemics, although at the time I felt I was making an obvious statement more than arguing a point. And in 1997 the modeling exercises of researchers Martina Morris and Mirjam Kretzschmar suggested that the final size of an HIV epidemic increases *exponentially* as the number of partners rises.[3] That is, instead of growing 1-2-3-4-5 and so on, it grows 1-2-4-8-16. This dynamic goes a long way to explaining why Uganda's self-designed public-health messages urging people to "be faithful" succeeded when so many other interventions have failed. We think fairly clearly about linear cause-and-effect, but networks are difficult to grasp. Indeed, their effects can be counterintuitive—one reason economic forecasts are so often wrong. Because fidelity breaks up sexual networks, it has a much stronger impact than one might expect. Morris and Kretzschmar showed that small decreases in the number of sexual partners could sometimes slash the size of networks.[4]

Imagine partner reduction as a scissors: cut the web at the right places and it fragments; each virus suddenly has a much smaller neighborhood. Or more linearly: Alice may infect Ben, but if Ben is faithful, Diane and Ellen don't get HIV and spread it further; infection rates therefore plunge. Let's take it to the ultimate. If each fragment has no more than two people—if everyone is totally monogamous—we have viral lockout. I could be the most promiscuous man since Don Juan, but if the women I seduced (and their husbands) were strict monogamists, I'd have zero risk of sexually transmitted HIV.

Networks also explain why delay of sexual debut matters. The period between loss of virginity and first marriage is especially dangerous for women.[5] In an Africa-wide ecological analysis of Demographic and Health Survey (DHS) data, demographer John Bongaarts found that sexually active women had more risk of exposure to HIV before the first marriage than after. His findings suggest that the size of African HIV epidemics is related to the number of years between first sex and marriage. The sooner women marry, the safer they are and the safer everyone is. Why? Husbands are more committed and less promiscuous. Premarriage women are inadvertently tapping into sexual networks, showing, as Bongaarts put it, the critical role of a high rate of new partner acquisition in the spread of epidemics.[6]

The Hazard Pyramid

I was in a taxi, en route to visit a South African who had recently written a dissertation called "Ideology and AIDS"—a dead-on title. En route I began to jot down in a notebook the different degrees of risk of HIV infection, depending on the type of relationship and the prevalence of networks. With several coauthors I ended up publishing a simple, heuristic typology of sexual relationships to guide thinking about appropriate behavioral interventions.[7] There are at least seven basic types of sexual partnerships worth considering, listed here in order of increasing risk, and each has subtypes reflecting "degree of":

1. Male and female in continuous monogamy
2. Male and female in serial monogamy with no partner overlap
3. Male and female in serial monogamy with partner overlap
4. Male and female, where the male has occasional nonregular partners, as with Asian or Latin American husbands who occasionally visit sex workers
5. Male and female, where the male has one concurrent partner, as with sugar daddies
6. Male and female, where each has a concurrent partner but the pattern is not usual in wider society (that is, they have little exposure to networks)
7. Male and female, where each has a concurrent partner and this pattern *is* usual in wider society (that is, they do face exposure to networks)

At each level we have a good idea of the factors that affect the risk. For example, at level 4—regular partnership with one person occasionally straying—the main risk factor is frequency of infidelity. How often does a husband go to the red-light district? At other levels the main risk factor may be how enduring the concurrent partner is, or the number of concurrent partners are. Each tier is a different audience for AIDS prevention messages. For example, couples in enduring relationships almost never use condoms. And it may well be harder to break up a years-long extramarital relationship than to prevent an occasional encounter with a sex worker, although research remains scanty here. So a one-size-fits-all approach misses most people.

The pyramid has no category for polygamy, an African custom in some places, but the crucial variable here is whether the union is an open or closed network. If it's closed, and all partners are HIV-negative, there is zero chance of sexually transmitted HIV. The fort is impregnable. But if the union is open to other partners, then everyone is at greater risk, in part because of the greater chance of encountering an HIV-positive partner in the early, ultracontagious phase.

$E^2 = (MC)^3$: The Circumcision Factor

Fidelity is not the whole story. Male circumcision also helps prevent AIDS. Investigators first noted a link between circumcision and lower infection rates around 1989, and my initial papers addressing it go back to 1992.[8] Since then, more than forty epidemiological studies, several meta-analyses, and randomized trials in South Africa, Kenya, and Uganda have probed this issue. The connection is clear and scarcely debated today. A 2002 UNAIDS study of four African cities found that male circumcision was one of the most important factors explaining HIV levels. (Condoms were without effect, a finding that had no impact on prevention policy. Instead, UNAIDS commissioned another study, which reached the same conclusion and went into the same drawer.[9]) In fact, cities with high circumcision rates had lower HIV prevalence even when sexual behavior patterns were similar. The first randomized trial of circumcision, held in South Africa, found that it can cut infection rates by 60 percent. Similar trials in Kenya and Uganda yielded similar findings.

The major organizations therefore geared up to roll out programs that promoted and made available voluntary male circumcision (already nicknamed "MC" by those of us working in this area). MC was a quick, simple outpatient operation, but epidemiological modelers pointed out that without fidelity, the 60 percent risk reduction could lead to "risk compensation" (more about this below) and higher HIV infection rates. Yet as I've seen so often in Africa, the outsiders overall lagged behind the people on the ground. I was aware by 1989 that MC might be protective, and in 1992 a traditional healer from Soweto told me that he routinely advised MC for his clients to prevent STDs. I tried to find out if he was a lone example. Several other healers strongly agreed that MC helped prevent STDs and even HIV, and they too had urged their clients to become circumcised. I collected anecdotal evidence that healers from societies that traditionally practiced MC (for example, Thonga, Xhosa) were advising people from noncircumcising societies (such as Zulu, Swazi) to become circumcised to help prevent STDs. The clients apparently were complying by visiting hospitals (not traditional healers) for the operation. I received a pamphlet dated 1991 and mass-produced by TRADAP (Traditional Doctors AIDS Project), one of the healers' organizations that had participated in the workshop. It advised: "To circumcise is the best remedy to reduce sexually transmitted diseases."

The scientific community would need another decade to catch on, however.[10] So how did the traditional healers spot this association so early, innocent as they were of the scientific literature? They told me it was because of their "clinical practice."[11] They could not fail to notice that the men who kept coming to them with STDs presented uncircumcised penises. What's more, adult men were reportedly taking the healers' advice and going to hospitals for circumcision. When I reported this fact to our USAID-funded project manager, suggesting that I follow up on these men and possibly do a randomized, controlled trial, I was told to back off. Forget it all and get back to condom promotion. So I had to settle for giving oral presentations at conferences, starting that same year, and publishing a letter in *Tropical Doctor* and later in *The Lancet*.[12]

Why does MC work? There seem to be several reasons. First, the foreskin is vulnerable to HIV. Its inner part abounds with Langerhans cells, which act as gateways for HIV into the body. In addition, the foreskin can tear, letting the bug directly into the blood, and the virus may be able to survive a while nestled under the organ, whereas it quickly dies on dry skin. Uncircumcised men are also more apt to have STDs like herpes and syphilis, as the healers observed, and the sores are portals for HIV. In 2007, after many attacks on the Uganda ABC model (abstain, be faithful, or use a condom) as "simplistic,"

I offered another formula, half in jest. I said: For those of you who say ABC is not complex enough, how about this?

$$E^2 = (MC)^3$$

Let me explain. HIV hyperEpidemics (E^2 rather than E) result from three things: Multiple Concurrent (partners), compounded by lack of Male Circumcision and (to make it more acceptable) Misuse or nonuse of Condoms. Understand? This formula avoids the fearsome A-word: abstinence. We actually held a conference in South Africa that December called "Beyond the $E^2 = (MC)^3$." I didn't choose the title, but it also slightly mocked the over-use of "Beyond the . . . ," as in "Beyond the ABCs," with its strong implication that ABC was something that had been tried and now we need to get beyond it.

It Wasn't Condoms

Let's take another look at why we are quite sure condoms didn't cause the AIDS drop-off in Uganda. Not only did *I* witness the inchoate distribution in 1993, but many scholars have documented the absence of condoms in the turnaround years. For instance, the 2006 study "How Uganda Reversed Its HIV Epidemic," concluded that "counseling and testing and condom promotion were very small elements in the early years in which the changes in seroprevalence [i.e., prevalence] were first seen."[13] Doug Kirby—an expert in adolescent sexual behavior about whom I'll speak considerably more later in this book—analyzed seven sources of evidence about Uganda in the early years: models of HIV prevalence and incidence, newspaper articles, written records of condom shipments, historical documents, and three kinds of surveys. He concluded that "all seven types of data produced consistent evidence that people in Uganda first reduced their number of sexual partners."[14] Similarly, Jim Shelton, a top adviser in the Office of Family Planning at USAID, and his colleague Beverly

Johnston investigated the average number of condoms available per male ages fifteen to nineteen in several African countries, over a ten-year period. During the unprecedented decline of HIV in Uganda from 1989 through 2000, there were only four condoms per male, per year.[15] Condom availability in Africa still remains very low, largely because of low "demand."

The early condom void helped make Ugandan president Museveni a skeptic. In a speech at a global AIDS conference in 1991, he said: "In countries like ours, where a mother often has to walk twenty miles to get an aspirin for her sick child or five miles to get any water at all, the practical questions of getting a constant supply of condoms or using them properly may never be resolved." And yet, he added: "We are being told that only a thin piece of rubber stands between us and the death of our continent." He noted that condoms might play some role, but they could hardly repel the tide of AIDS alone.

Museveni was not invited to another major global AIDS conference until 2004.

It *Couldn't* Have Been Condoms

What if the West had acted faster and saturated Uganda with condoms early on, putting them on every street corner and giving them away for free? Even then the devices could not have cut back the epidemic. Why not? If condoms were ubiquitous and people worried about dying, how could they *not* have helped? The argument for condoms sounds appealing, partly because we can easily see how they work. The latex simply blocks the virus, as a glass dome will hold in bees. However, the process requires further steps that we too often fail to visualize. A single use by one couple must extend to consistent use by that couple—and then to consistent use by *all* couples. So it's a snap to think that because condoms block the virus, everyone would be safe if they just used them. Networks wouldn't matter, because the virus couldn't get in.

Unfortunately, reality intervenes on all three levels: (1) condoms can fail in a single use; (2) the great majority of users don't use them consistently; and (3) most people won't use them at all, despite persistent efforts dating back long before HIV.

First, condoms aren't virus-proof. In a single use they can leak, break, and slip. Partners can deploy them improperly in the heat of passion, especially if they have been drinking. Even if worn every time, condoms provide only an 80 to 85 percent reduction in risk (compared to those who don't use condoms at all), over a period of usually a year, according to an oft-cited meta-analysis.[16] Risk of infection is also cumulative, growing greater with passage of time, assuming contact with HIV-infected partners. The 80 to 85 percent risk reduction is under ideal conditions, meaning that these data come from highly motivated people: "discordant" couples (one has HIV and the other doesn't) who have received both condoms and counseling.

How well do condoms work in the real world of Africa? A careful Johns Hopkins study in Uganda, in a population better informed and supplied than most, found that condoms reduced risk by only 65 percent.[17] Overall, Africa poses special problems for condom safety. I once spent a day interviewing people at a sweltering clinic in the rural Qwa-Qwa area of South Africa, in the twilight of the apartheid era. Short of furniture, the clinic had turned full crates of condoms into tables and chairs. The condoms had come from Thailand and they were unusable because they were "Asian-sized" (the other end of the spectrum from "African-sized," not to add further to stereotypes). Moreover, storage in heat can harm rubbers and cause them to break, and they were probably deteriorating here. It happens all over Africa. Storage past the expiration date is also common and likewise causes rupture. The matron of the clinic commented that "someone" was sending too many crates of condoms, more than they could even give away.

A raft of other defects has appeared in highly infected countries.

In 2002, for example, Tanzania forbade a UN agency from import-
ing ten million condoms after lab tests found defects, and in 2007
South Africa recalled twenty million of them. In 2009 major condom brands failed safety tests in Zambia and Kenya. In 2004, after
Ugandans complained that a popular brand showed signs of deg-
radation, the government withdrew it. The brand lost public trust,
and in 2007 Uganda reported that forty million of these devices
were likely to expire because of low demand. In every case people
discovered these problems before distribution—that is, before heat
could go to work.

Nonetheless, companies market condoms as if they are near-
perfect. One article in the *Times of Zambia*, written in the name of
a local condom organization, told readers: "According to the WHO,
condoms are up to 97 per cent effective when used correctly and
consistently, i.e., properly every time you have sex. The failure rate
is mainly due to the fact that people do not use condoms every time
they have sex or do not learn how to use them properly."[18] These
extravagant claims are widespread and come from condom social
marketers, whose salaries and career advancement often depend on
how many condoms they have "moved." I speak as a former condom
social marketer.

Second, it's hard to get couples to use condoms consistently. Think of
a discordant couple that decides to rely on condoms. It's not enough
to use them now and then. The partners have to use them consistently. In a ten-year study in Rakai, Uganda, researchers found that
consistent condom use reduced risk of HIV infection by 63 percent,
yet inconsistent use had no effect at all—even after adjusting for
demographic and behavioral variables (such as the tendency for
inconsistent users to have more partners and riskier sex). This is a
serious finding, because irregular use is so common. In this study
4.4 percent of the population reported consistent condom use over
the past year and 16.5 percent inconsistent use.[19] In plain language:

most condom use is inconsistent and inconsistent use does not protect against AIDS.

In fact, intermittent use may correlate with greater chance of
infection. A study of South African youth concluded that it was a
significant risk behavior for HIV infection.[20] There, 19.7 percent of
young men and 16.6 percent of young women reported consistent
use—much fewer than those reporting condom use at *last* intercourse, by the way—and sporadic users of both sexes were more apt
to get HIV than nonusers. A study of military draftees in Thailand
has also shown a link between irregular condom use and a higher
rate of STDs. The consequences of inconsistent use need further
investigation. Unfortunately, it's been difficult so far. Most surveys
ask only about condom use at most recent sex, and this "last use"
statistic can be misleading. Imagine a population where each man
used a condom at *every other* act of intercourse. On-off-on-off—and so
on. The last-use tally would be 50 percent, suggesting that 50 percent
of men used condoms consistently and 50 percent never used them
at all. In fact, everyone would be using condoms and no one would
be using them consistently. Hence reported increases in condom use
may not reflect any real reduction in risk.

Even discordant couples don't use condoms as regularly as we
might expect. Despite the obvious threat to life, in Rwanda only nine
of fifty-three discordant couples reported using condoms every time.[21]
In Zambia researchers followed discordant couples for a year and did
biological tests to verify the self-reports. About a fourth of the couples
said they had been consistent users over each of the following periods:
(a) the past year, (b) three of the past four quarters, (c) two of the past
four, and (d) one or none of them. Researchers found sperm in vaginal smears in 15 percent of the "consistent use" individuals, so the
couples overestimated their consistency. Intriguingly, even consistent
use was associated with only a 52 percent reduction in HIV transmission. In a very recent, breakthrough analysis of DHS data from four

African countries, we found no correlation at all between consistent use and HIV levels—that is, a person who at least reported always using a condom was just as likely to have HIV as one who never did.

Third, people don't use condoms. At the whole-population level condoms have always been a Hail Mary strategy: if only, if only, if only. And the hoped-for condition has always been clear. Look at Thailand as an example. Condom promoters declare it the world's greatest condom success story. In the 1990s prostitutes in its famous sex industry began requiring customers to wear latex and a decline in HIV soon appeared. Its incidence dropped during the early part of the decade, and prevalence fell from 2 percent in 1995 to 1.6 percent in 2001, according to tests on pregnant women at antenatal clinics. So why can't we just import the Thai strategy to Africa? For one thing, Thailand had a concentrated epidemic rather than a generalized one. The locus lay with sex workers, and during the early 1990s the percentage of customers who used condoms consistently with prostitutes almost doubled, rising from 36 percent to 71 percent.

Even there, however, condoms alone were not responsible. By the end of the early 1990s far fewer Thai customers were entering the red-light districts. Indeed, male traffic to sex workers dropped by half, from 22 percent to 10 percent in a national sample. Male premarital and extramarital sex in general also fell by half.[22] But this behavior change was almost always ignored by the time I started to challenge the constant references to the success of the 100 percent condom-use policy in Thailand, and the claims that we could just transplant it anywhere.

In Africa, AIDS doesn't radiate out from a clear center, and only 1.6 percent of Ugandan men reported paying for sex during the past year, according to recent DHS data. Such men may use condoms, but they are not a major factor in the epidemic. The virus is everywhere in major parts of Africa, so the meaningful condom figures are those for the population. In 1995 about one in sixteen sexually active Ugandans used a condom with some regularity, according to the DHS. By 2000 this proportion had risen to one in nine of the sexually active, or one in twelve of all Ugandans. Condom use has become quite high among those at high risk, the relatively few who are still having multiple partners (for example, 59 percent of men with nonmarital, noncohabiting partners, and over 95 percent among sex workers and their clients—very close to the user rates found among prostitutes in Thailand). But if we look at DHS results for "condom use, last sex, any partner, of those sexually active," we see that condom use is actually lower in Uganda than in many other countries in the region.

The problem lies less in distribution than demand, and demand is slack in Africa for many of the reasons found everywhere. For one thing, using a condom with a steady partner has serious trust implications. It says, "I think you could be unfaithful to me." People simply don't want to send that message, or even think it. Condoms also decrease male pleasure and require an awkward break in love-making. They aren't user-friendly. How hard is it to get people to use condoms? Let's look at Thailand again. By 1996 nearly 90 percent of Bangkok sex workers were using rubbers, yet only 28.5 percent used them with nonpaying sex partners, such as boyfriends. They knew they were at high risk, yet three-quarters of them spurned the protection. Why did the percentages differ so much? Brothel owners could compel condom use, and did, under government pressure. But back in their apartments, prostitutes and their partners made their own decisions. And in the general population, condom use was even less common. Only 18.9 percent of women overall reported using rubbers at last sex.

There is also significant evidence that condoms protected custom-ers, not prostitutes. According to a study of Cambodian sex workers, "Despite the implementation of a nationwide 100 percent condom use policy, the prevalence of STIs [sexually transmitted infections] among female sex workers in 2005 was comparable to 2001."[23] Simi-larly, reported condom use among sex workers in Kampala rose to more than 90 percent by the early 2000s, yet HIV infection rates among them still climbed. Why? The likely reason is that the men have far fewer exposures. In any case, today we can no longer say the "Thai model" is working in Thailand (or anywhere else). Things are not going well there. Sex work has greatly increased, much of it has moved out of the bordellos, and condom use has dropped off. It is hard to be sure that HIV is actually rising in Thailand, given the unreliability of figures before 2007. However, gay men now account for a fifth of all infections, and in Bangkok HIV prevalence among them rose from 17 percent in 2003 to 28 percent in 2005. Among younger gay men HIV prevalence tripled over the same three-year period. In 2005 married women accounted for more than 30 percent of the new HIV cases. According to the *Bangkok Post*, citing Dr. Sombat Tanprasertsuk, director of the AIDS, Tuberculosis, and Sexually Transmitted Diseases Bureau in Thailand: "Lack of abstinence, faithfulness and condom use (ABC) was the major cause of the increase in the infection rate among married women."[24]

In Africa further factors mute demand for condoms. For instance, many people fear that potent sexual fluids could fall into the hands of sorcerers and other evil-doers. Condoms have a different history in Africa than in the West or, say, in Thailand. Their prime function has always been to curb venereal disease, not to limit the number of children. Hence they have a somewhat lurid aura, associated with profligacy and prostitution. In 2007, South African serial rapist Mongezi Jingxela told police: "I've never used a condom. The problem is that where I grew up, these items were highly forbidden." Of course we don't expect such criminals to use condoms, but it is intriguing to hear the rapist of at least seventy-one women base his decision on conservative community values.

The fact is, no one has ever found a way to get people in a general population to use condoms. Yet the lure endlessly beckons, enticing donors year after year. Thus, after a quarter century of relentless promotion, UNAIDS in its "Letter to Partners 2010" could still write:

"In sub-Saharan Africa, only four condoms were available each year for every adult male of reproductive age." The average was slightly over four a decade earlier. According to a study in the *British Medical Journal*, condom levels peaked in sub-Saharan Africa in the mid-1990s. So as AIDS went on to explode in southern Africa, reaching the highest levels ever seen on earth, condom provision and possibly condom demand remained stable for Africa as a whole, or actually declined somewhat. Those I debate cite the same statistics as an argument to do more, to supply more.

Despite the foregoing, I support condom use for those who cannot or will not be careful (or who know or suspect their partners won't). They clearly have an effect one-on-one, and in Thailand and Cambodia, where bordello owners could compel their use, condoms plus behavior change smothered an AIDS epidemic. But in Africa the disease hides everywhere, and condoms are just a backup. They are no substitute for low-risk behavior.

Back in the Dominican Republic

Once I saw the Uganda success in combating the spread of AIDS, I began to look for similar evidence elsewhere, including the DR, where I had had my first fifteen minutes of fame back in 1988. In 1998, I returned to conduct behavioral research there. ProFamilia, the affiliate of International Planned Parenthood Association, had asked me to come back to help figure out why reported condom use had leveled off and may have been declining. Of course, the first thing that occurred to me was that precisely because of the DR's early success in raising AIDS awareness, men might be switching to fidelity—because it's inherently safer than continuing to visit sex workers, even with condoms. The more fidelity, the less need for condoms.

We did a quick survey, using a low-cost national representative sample, and we happened to be in the field at roughly the same time as the DHS. Comparing answers to similar or identical questions in the two surveys, our findings were within the margin of error, suggesting our sampling and methods were good. (And, gratifyingly, our survey cost about five thousand dollars, apart from my consultancy. The DHS study cost about one million dollars.) We found that Dominican men indeed seemed to be shifting to fidelity. This news was major. Not only was the DR's program continuing to succeed, but we had further evidence that fidelity was a practical way to block the AIDS virus.

But my family-planning colleagues and USAID were not happy with our findings; I was never again invited back to the DR. One journal after another turned down an article we wrote based on our survey. In a high moment for the scientific method, some peer reviewers stated outright that my Dominican coauthor and I were dangerous, anticondom ideologues whom no one should ever publish. Several reviewers stated that condoms were our best weapon against AIDS, as if this notion were established fact. I then tried submitting the article to anthropology journals, but to no avail. Editors trying to be helpful suggested I might want to rewrite the article from scratch and weave in a theme of interest to anthropologists, such as women's empowerment, stigma, homophobia, or the role of poverty in driving AIDS. Apparently, driving down the infection rate was a theme of no more interest to anthropologists than to medical or public-health journals. My coauthor and I finally managed to find a receptive journal editor, and we squeezed our findings into a tiny letter.[25]

Well, paradigm shifts take time. Throughout the 1990s I believed AIDS experts would soon catch up with ever-accumulating evidence and do the right thing. They *had* to, because more and more Africans were suffering every day. I repeatedly stated that I was not trying to replace condoms. I wanted to add strategies that were conspicuously absent: discouraging people from having multiple partners and postponing debut. Otherwise, people would think they could have as many sex partners as they liked, as long as they wore a condom. I was saying, OK, let's keep doing what we have been doing, but now that we have far more funds than we ever believed possible, exploding from tens to hundreds of millions per year (and to seven *billion* annually by 2007), let's not just put new money in the exact same place as old money. Let's also try something new, something like Uganda did. But no. It would take nearly another decade to find cracks in the fortress.

And the Award Goes to . . .

Meanwhile, the media and the world were told that condoms were the key to the Uganda achievement. A 2000 *Newsweek* cover story about the horror of AIDS in Africa pointed out that there was at least one success story to learn from: Uganda. "In Uganda," the magazine told its readers, "health workers turned Protector condoms into must-have fashion accessories, simply by introducing a flashy new package and a marketing slogan ('So strong, so smooth')." The piece mentioned no other prevention method. Of course, reporters only know what AIDS experts tell them. Academic papers are still appearing that try to make the case that condoms are responsible for Uganda's HIV decline, although most peer-reviewed articles since 2005 that analyze Uganda's success have started to get that one story basically right.

"I look at condoms as an improvisation, not a solution," President Museveni told delegates on the second day of the Fifteenth International AIDS Conference in Bangkok in 2004. Instead, he called for "optimal relationships based on love and trust instead of institutionalized mistrust, which is what the condom is all about." CNN used his speech as an opportunity to poll its viewers around the globe. However, it recast Museveni's approach as abstinence and asked viewers whether they agreed or disagreed with it as the best solution to African AIDS. Surprise: most viewers disagreed. This particular confusion has been widespread for decades. But it's the difference between void and presence. Abstinence is sex with no one. Fidelity is sex with one person. One is rare and difficult, and the other is the most common sexual relationship on earth.

CHAPTER 5

Infidelity

Uganda's success had been astonishing. A simple, home-grown program cut the HIV prevalence by two-thirds, from 15 percent to 5 percent. A tiny, impoverished African nation reeling from decades of cruelty had notched one of the greatest public-health achievements in history. And then, as I predicted in my 2003 book, *Rethinking AIDS Prevention*, the disease started crawling back. The dive in measures of HIV prevalence ended around 2004, and the DHS in 2005 showed it to be 6.7 percent, considerably higher than previously estimated. Other data suggested a rise in new infections. An ongoing study in the Rakai district revealed that HIV incidence started trending upward in 2003. Another study, based on data from 203,000 voluntary counseling and testing (VCT) clients examined between 1993 and 2003, found that annual HIV incidence per 100 uninfected persons increased from 0.9 in 1993 to 2.3 in 2003.

What was going on? It seemed an enigma, so a variety of explanations emerged. Two of the most prominent were: (1) people weren't using enough condoms, and (2) the Bush administration had foisted too much abstinence upon Ugandans. Human Rights Watch released a report in March 2005 which claimed that Uganda was abandoning condoms in favor of an "abstinence-only" strategy, and published a widely distributed article entitled "Uganda: 'Abstinence-Only' Programs Hijack AIDS Success Story." Uganda's purported change in strategy was even discussed in the U.S. Congress and in the Institute of Medicine's later evaluation of the Bush administration's African AIDS bill, known as PEPFAR.

Those of us not fond of Bush and his administration found it tempting to blame its policies. However, the evidence points elsewhere. Ugandan officials have dismissed the Human Rights Watch claim as nonsense, and indeed the recent trend has been toward more condom use, not less. In fact, by about 2004, Uganda's anti-AIDS program had blended in with those in the rest of Africa. Instead of the failures mimicking the lone success, the success was taking lessons from the failures, with their expensive condom social marketing, supplemented by STD treatment, and attempts at HIV testing. At the same time, disturbingly, the DHS showed that people were having more multiple partners again. The broken sexual networks were reforming. Since the mid-1990s the proportion of men and women reporting multiple partners has increased—from 1 percent to 4 percent of women, and from 10 percent to 28 percent for men. The results were unnerving but inevitable, as I warned in a 2004 letter published in the *New York Times:* HIV would rise again in the World Great AIDS Success Story, thanks to *us.*[1]

The Lost Message

You could see the difference in the streets. One member of the Uganda AIDS Commission (UAC), after describing the central role of fidelity and delay in Uganda's HIV decline, mentioned that "behavior change" messages had somehow dwindled away since the early 1990s: "We sometimes see faded billboards that used to have AIDS messages. Now they just have messages about condoms or Coke." Recently, University of California epidemiologist Norman Hearst, researchers from Makerere University in Kampala, and I carried out studies revealing direct evidence of changes in people's attitudes. In March and April 2009 we conducted interviews and focus groups in a low-income urban outskirt area of Kampala and in a rural village outside Kampala. The urban area was the same one where Hearst and some of his Ugandan colleagues had conducted an earlier study showing that increased condom use correlated with greater HIV risk.[2]

As this book goes to press, preliminary findings yield an unsettling picture. When asked to rank the effectiveness of prevention methods, both men and women put testing for HIV status first, followed by condoms. Significantly down the list came fidelity, and abstinence ranked last. We then asked, "Over the last six months what is the main AIDS message you have heard or seen?" Three-quarters of men and women answered testing or condoms. The survey also found that 95 percent of women and 98 percent of men said they knew where to get a condom if they needed one. No one mentioned "zero grazing" or "love faithfully"—the two most remembered slogans in the 1991 USAID baseline survey. Thus attitudes have switched from favoring behavior change to testing and condoms.

Of course, other changes in viewpoint likely undermined Uganda's AIDS fortunes as well. Our study also found ample evidence that people have come to see AIDS as a treatable, chronic disease like malaria. In other words the availability of antiretrovirals (ARVs) has lowered their fear of it, a downside I warned about in my 2003 book. (And of course I wholeheartedly support these life-preserving drugs. Indeed, I would have used my own money to save my friend Joe.) Ugandans no longer see AIDS victims wasting away before their eyes. Many respondents made comments about disinhibition, such as, "Ever since people began getting ARVs, they have had irresponsible sex. They're not afraid they might infect each other with the AIDS virus." Some "prevention fatigue" was likely inevitable too. A country cannot stay on high alert forever, and it was probably unrealistic to expect the widespread feelings of vulnerability and caution of the late 1980s to continue. But Uganda's adoption of the global prevention standard—testing and condoms—and its turn away from behavior change probably sealed its fate.

We see why people's attitudes might have changed. In 2004 the newspaper *The Monitor* ran an article by unnamed "AIDS activists" who claimed there was no evidence that fidelity or delay lowered HIV rates. However, the article said, condom use had risen as HIV infections fell, seesaw-like. The piece featured a photo of the minister of health, giving the impression that he endorsed its conclusions. The authors seemed unaware that while condom use rose in Uganda, it increased even more in other African countries, where HIV infections were rising to even higher levels. They also seemed ignorant of the UNAIDS finding that promoting condoms to the general population seems associated with increased HIV rates.

But it wasn't just the media. The shift in public attitude, it turned out, stemmed from official policy. The Ugandan government itself had made the U-turn.

Fidelity and the Strategy Frameworks

I have tried to reconstruct the history of when and how Uganda drifted from its original ABC program to the condom-oriented one. I have looked at "The National Strategic Framework for HIV/AIDS Activities in Uganda for 2000/1–2005/6," which I got from the Ugandan government. It was written by the Uganda AIDS Commission, with support from USAID. The framework is a huge thirty-one-page-long matrix that details objectives, intermediate results, sectors involved, activities, impact indicators, and results. I first saw the report in 2001, when I was part of a team to help the USAID mission in Uganda plan its HIV/AIDS activities for the next five years. (Incidentally, the USAID mission kept our final design document in pre-acceptance limbo for more than a year. Two things I suspect they didn't like were that we gave credit to ABC—especially fidelity—for Uganda's success, and we also gave credit to the Ugandan government, as distinct from just the NGO sector, for developing this turnaround strategy.)

Interestingly, "faithfulness" appeared only twice in the matrix, both times merely in a passing statement of a general goal of "abstinence, faithfulness and condoms." Yet the word "condom" appeared twenty-nine times, and not just in passing. The document laid out specific objectives and indicators for the devices, such as "increase condom accessibility and affordability with particular emphasis to rural areas," and "train communities based distribution agents (CBDs) on condom distribution practices, and establish condom distribution networks in rural areas." Likewise, there were measures of success, such as (a) the number of condom distribution outlets set up in rural and urban areas; (b) the percentage of sexually active rural residents who said they could get condoms easily; and (c) the percentage of men, women, and youth who said they used condoms consistently and correctly. But nowhere in this 2001 strategic-planning document was there an objective related to fidelity or delay. Three years later, the same was true for the updated document.

Objectives and impact indicators are essential, because the people who implement programs are responsible for reaching the objectives, as measured by the impact indicators. If all indicators relate to condoms and drugs, no fidelity activities will occur. I happen to have an even earlier strategy framework from Uganda, given to me by the Ugandan government in 1998. "Condom" comes up less frequently, only thirteen times. And in the objectives column, both "mutual faithfulness" and "encourage the norm of having fewer sexual partners" appear as goals for sexually active people over age twenty. "Abstinence until marriage" and "delayed onset of 1st sexual activity" also appear here. Again, these objectives all had vanished by 2001. Earlier national planning documents dating back to 1993 are full of targets and impact indicators for fidelity and abstinence. All of which raises the question of why Uganda would have dismantled a program it knew had saved the lives of perhaps a million of its citizens—that is, more than the number who died in the nearby Rwandan genocide.

Visitors from the West

I returned to Uganda in 2004, when the nation was again developing its National Strategic Plan, and the situation was bleak. Indeed, I was pretty sure Uganda's fidelity initiative would not survive. It wasn't yet clear that prevalence had increased, but in an e-mail to my colleagues and supporters I wrote at the time: "When condomization of this program reaches a certain point (which in fact may already have been reached), HIV prevalence will rise again and the ABC critics will say, 'See! ABC never worked! We need to bring condom levels up to those of Botswana!'" What caused the difference? I believe Vinand Nantulya, a Ugandan physician and immunology researcher, was right when he said that Uganda had been lucky that it had no foreign AIDS experts when the epidemic struck. "People used their own wisdom to curb the spread of the epidemic," he said. "The president just captured the common thinking of the people."[3]

But then the foreign HIV advisers appeared, and they began telling Ugandans that fidelity and abstinence didn't work. Science had proven it, they said. Moreover, they added, both strategies spread stigma and disempowered women. These foreigners had the world's most successful AIDS program right before their eyes yet they couldn't see it. One American AIDS adviser from a major university told me in front of a Ugandan health educator that "Ugandans are the most promiscuous people in the world." I asked why therefore such high percentages of Ugandans reported fidelity or abstinence on the most recent Demographic and Health Survey. She was unaware of this fact. Most Ugandans knew better, so why didn't they speak up? Some did, of course, but it's hard for Westerners to imagine the situation there. Outside donors are the sugar daddies of AIDS policy. They pay for everything. As travel writer Paul Theroux correctly observed, in rural Africa donors seem about the only people with money and their presence warps the whole economy.

For example, the 2007 National Strategic Plan for AIDS will cost $2 billion over five years—an incredible sum for Uganda, whose annual government revenues are $2.6 billion. (Of that $2 billion, about $75 million—less than 4 percent—was allotted to behavior change, the only strategy that will save a substantial number of lives.) And because foreign donors will pay almost all of this bill, the local AIDS industry is likely one of the top foreign exchange sources in the country. The great disparity in power and resources means that Ugandans (indeed, most Africans) cannot easily stand up and defend the most effective AIDS prevention program the world has ever known. Many Ugandan intellectuals and AIDS officials know what is going on, but they have too much at stake: their salaries, often their cars, funding for their specific programs, international travel (where even a few weeks of per diems can be worth more than regular annual salaries for civil servants), and even easy access to life-saving medications. (Many Ugandans are HIV-positive and obtained these drugs before their fellow citizens.) To advance their careers, they play the game, and the donors define the ground rules. Ugandans either go along or find other employment.

Of course, flooding a poor African country with cash invites abuse. And a major scandal did break out in Uganda in 2006. The Uganda Judicial Commission of Inquiry learned that an array of officials, from top government ministers to ordinary community workers, had been embezzling from the $45.3 million given to Uganda from the Global Fund to Fight AIDS, Tuberculosis, and Malaria. Six months later, a government white paper agreed, aggressive prosecution of several government officials was urged; the report declared that the malefactors should repay at least $1.6 million. The minister of health had to resign, and in April 2009 one man was sentenced to ten years in jail. The affair was a dramatic humiliation for the nation that had pioneered effective AIDS prevention.

The Data Gap

The imbalance was not just a matter of money. There was a big data disparity as well. The natural advocates for fidelity and abstinence, the religious and other values-based leaders, were unfamiliar with the behavioral or serological data. In fact, they assumed the scientists and activists knew that information, and so by default they fell back on moral arguments. This fact has made them easy to discredit. Indeed, almost all recognized AIDS experts dismissed African questioning of condoms and drugs as uneducated, religiously motivated moralizing. They framed the issue as one of scientific understanding versus pious dogma. All of this helped nourish the "best and the brightest" mentality among these policymakers, a sense of intellectual superiority like that among JFK and Lyndon Johnson's advisers during the Vietnam War.

Funders therefore lauded the best Ugandan condom promoters as "progressive" and "enlightened"—that is, ahead of the slower minds. Indeed, some Ugandans have actually come to believe in condoms and drugs. And why wouldn't they? Many have received education in America or Europe and heard lessons from the top experts in global AIDS and reproductive health. Or they have been sent abroad for short courses. Or they have read the medical journals. All of this exposure reinforces this specific belief, despite the firsthand experience in their own country. And the data-rich misinformation in Uganda wasn't cheap. A 2002 USAID report observed: "Total donor support for all AIDS-related contributions during the period 1989–1998 was approximately $180 million, or about $1.80 per adult per year over the 10-year period."[4] That's eight times as much as before, and it was a trickle compared to the torrent to come.

Revolt

At the time of my 1998 visit to Uganda, these events lay in the future, but I could see them coming like the storm on a TV weather map.

Western attitudes and influence on AIDS were permeating Africa and suffocating the great lesson of Uganda. So I began speaking out about what was wrong with AIDS prevention, especially in Africa. I didn't have to be a telepath to realize that others deemed me politically incorrect in the extreme, a menace to a burgeoning industry. I couldn't get my articles on AIDS accepted, after a long career of publishing articles across several disciplinary boundaries. My paper for the World Bank, the fruit of my 1998 trip, vanished into the Bank's deep recesses and would not see daylight again. I gave spirited talks to top people in the industry, such as those at the Population Council, explaining that we had cheaper and truly effective ways to bring down the African death toll. They heard me out in cool silence.

Over the years I had kept waiting for someone to step up to the plate, say, some leading specialist in epidemiology and biostatistics. The pretense was clear and I knew I couldn't be the only one who saw through it. But no one else seemed to be stepping up. One day in 2001, I was sitting at my desk at home in Washington, D.C., poring over the official list of program impact indicators that USAID used to measure progress in AIDS prevention. The longer I looked at the list, the more indignant I became. *All* the measurements were about latex, drugs, or testing. As far as USAID was concerned, sexual behavior mattered as much as the breeze. Yet millions of Ugandans lay in their graves simply because they had had multiple and (probably) concurrent sex partners.

I decided at once to launch a jihad against the AIDS establishment. That's the actual word that came to mind: "jihad." Holy war. I swore to myself I would take on all of AIDS World and devote all my energies henceforth to exposing its pretenses. Whatever it took to dispel the falsehoods and reveal the truth, I would do it, by God! In righteous pique I hastily drafted a book proposal. If the scholarly community wouldn't let my ideas get past peer review, I'd do an end run and write a book. In fact, I realized that there was so much to expose, I'd need a book to do it. I Googled "academic publishers,"

chose ten among the names that popped up, and fired off my proposal to all of them, along with my full curriculum vitae. This entire
experience took about ninety minutes. Then I simmered down a bit
and went to the kitchen to make a salad for dinner and tell my wife
we were now in a holy war.

Over the next few weeks, to my surprise, I got two acceptances
and one "maybe." I decided to go with the best known house, Praeger. A week or so after the signing, I received a very modest check
in the mail. An advance! I had never gotten an advance before. It
never occurred to me to try to negotiate for one. A book advance
surely put me in the same category as Updike and Dostoevsky! I
was on a crusade. Even then I didn't quite understand the scale of
what I was battling.

PART III

CALAMITY'S CRADLE

The greatest blunders, like the thickest ropes, are often compounded of a multitude of strands.

VICTOR HUGO
Les Misérables

Sixty years of countless reform schemes to aid agencies and dozens of different plans, and $2.3 trillion later, the aid industry is still failing to reach the beautiful goal. The evidence points to an unpopular conclusion: Big Plans will always fail to reach the beautiful goal.

WILLIAM EASTERLY
The White Man's Burden

CHAPTER 6

Putting the Bedroom before the Sickroom

The global AIDS community promoted condoms in Africa despite the evidence. We banned fear appeals. We stayed mum about the risky behaviors that enflamed the pandemic—to the point that some South Africans thought most AIDS came from blood transfusions. We were undoing the spectacular success in Uganda. Why was this happening? Could the answer, I wondered, be something as simple as ideology?

In 1960 the sociologist Daniel Bell published *The End of Ideology*, whose title recalls Mark Twain's jest about reports of his death. Ideologies will always be with us, and the list of them keeps growing. But you don't often see ideology about the means to fight deadly epidemics. Yet that's exactly what I was seeing. Ideologies do exist on scientific issues, such as evolution and climate change; however, in these cases the ideologues are usually not scientists. With African AIDS, they often were.

As I traced back the chain of events, I realized that the ideology of sexual freedom was born from the conflict between rising wealth and traditional customs. As Western society grew richer in the nineteenth and early twentieth centuries, and innovations like the telephone and the automobile appeared, people had greater sexual opportunities, like the more affluent citizens in Africa today. They strained against the reigning strictures, and as a result controversies flared around the first "sexologists"—such as the Austro-German psychiatrist Richard Kraft-Ebing, the sex-centered opus of Sigmund Freud, and the novels of authors like D. H. Lawrence. Like a dam springing leaks here and there, the urge toward greater sexual freedom had multiple manifestations. Yet the evidence for its desirability could be illusion. For instance, the painter Paul Gauguin mythologized his life in the South Seas for folks back home, who spread the vision because it appealed to them. Other errors came from my own field of anthropology.

The Dream of Samoa

In 1926 anthropologist Margaret Mead stepped off a boat in Pago Pago, and two years later Western bookstores were showcasing her *Coming of Age in Samoa*. This ethnographic study became a best seller and, indeed, a national conversation piece. And no wonder. Mead, a smart, diminutive, and delightful scientist—I met her once in Pittsburgh—described a society in which young girls grew up with complete sexual freedom. "The concept of celibacy is absolutely meaningless to them," she declared. Hence they had "no confusion about sex" and "no woes."[1] In other words, sexual freedom brightened society. It could make people happier and more fulfilled, and liberate them from needless anxiety. By extension, culture had repressed sexuality in the West and stunted our lives. These conclusions swept across the world and had long-lasting influence. At Mead's death in 1978, *Coming of Age in Samoa* was still selling a hundred thousand copies a year.

But was she right? In 1983 the New Zealand anthropologist Derek Freeman challenged her conclusions in his *Margaret Mead and the Heretic*.[2] The anthropologist, he said, had not done her research. For instance, she had never seemed to notice that young Samoan women weren't getting pregnant before marriage. Incredibly, she acquired most of her "data" from a pair of adolescent girls, who got nervous and giggly under this intrusive interrogation and cooked up wild stories about unrestrained sex under a tropical moon. After all, that's what the strange white woman clearly wanted to hear. We anthropologists now call this institutionalized prevarication, a mechanism whereby those on the lower side of unequal power relationships present spurious depictions of their customs to outsiders, to protect themselves. Mead also concluded—based on a single conversation with a single Samoan schoolteacher—that there was no neurosis, no frigidity, no impotence in Samoa. All that teen sex makes us neurosis-free. Certainly my own Free Love generation would be quick to accept this idea. This male informant later wrote his own book depicting very different behavioral patterns in his culture.[3]

An academic brouhaha ensued over just how sexually liberated—or different from ourselves—Samoans actually were. Even though Freeman obviously spoke far better Samoan than Mead, and had done much more detailed, comprehensive, and scientific fieldwork in Samoa, he faced a sea of angry feminists, sexologists, and anthropologists who were upset at this mud on the icon. A good part of the backlash was over timing: why did Freeman wait until Mead's death to refute her findings? Freeman tried to publish his criticism of Mead's work as early as 1971, but his first manuscript was rejected by American editors, according to his obituary in the New York Times. A foundation rock of the sexual revolution was found cracked. The debate continues today, remarkably, but clearly Freeman was basically right. Samoa has well-defined sexual mores, and female virginity was in fact highly valued and usually practiced. By 2010 the nation had around 20 people living with HIV out of a population of 220,000, and so obviously very few sexual networks. We would have to look elsewhere for carnal Shangri-La.

Mead's mentor was another famous anthropologist, Ruth Benedict. Both of them—and their own mentor "Papa" Franz Boas, the father of American anthropology—were out to show that culture was far more important than biology. This position was courageous in the 1920s, when racism and fascism prevailed, but the two women perhaps wanted to please Papa Franz a little too much. What could prove the primacy of culture more bracingly than a discovery that gender roles were little more than cultural constructions? Indeed, after Samoa, Mead went on to discover a Melanesian tribe where the women allegedly did all the work, while men sat around gossiping and trying out hairstyles in mirrors. I heard somebody mention this finding again recently at a conference in South Africa, using nearly the same language I had heard in freshman sociology. Mysteriously, no other exotic tribe has been found where gender roles are so reversed. Psychologist Steven Pinker wrote of Mead in 1997: "She said that the Tshambuli reversed our sex roles, the men wearing curls and makeup. In fact the men beat their wives, exterminated neighboring tribes, and treated homicide as a milestone in a young man's life which entitled him to wear the face paint that Mead thought was so effeminate."[4]

The Hidden Libertines

After World War II, in 1948 and 1953, biology professor Alfred Kinsey issued a pair of reports on sex in America that also became best sellers. In anonymous surveys he found surprising levels of homosexuality, extramarital sex, childhood sex, and other practices most people thought were rather uncommon. For instance, he wrote that a judge, facing a defendant charged with a homosexual act, "should keep in mind that nearly 40 per cent of the males in the town could be arrested on similar charges at some time in their lives for similar activity," adding that the local police, court officials, clergy, and businessmen all have the same high rates of homosexuality.[5] A reviewer in *The Nation* digested Kinsey's findings for the public. They showed "that 85 percent of American males have pre-marital intercourse; . . . that from 30 to 45 percent have extra-marital intercourse; that 37 percent have had some homosexual experience; and that 17 percent of farm boys have intercourse with animals." The book critic added: "These figures may be slightly changed by further studies, but on the whole they would appear to be accurate—and they come as no surprise to anyone who has intimate and undistorted knowledge of human relations." His ultimate conclusion was simple: "A happy and harmonious sexual life is the greatest asset an individual can have, and the best guaranty of a powerful and benign social structure."[6]

The worldly reviewer for *The Nation* aside, these statistics didn't jibe with most people's sense of the world. Yet Kinsey was tallying closed-door behaviors. Who could tell? Maybe he was right. In fact, scholars have now largely discredited Kinsey's studies. He was a hyperactive bisexual who pressured his wife into joining group sex, and in his samples he deliberately sought unconventional respondents, recruiting men in prisons, group sex parties, and gay hangouts, so his reports greatly exaggerated the extent of unusual sex.[7] Outlying behaviors were just that, and not very common in America. He had violated the fundamental rule of survey research: use a random sample. Imagine, for instance, doing a survey of your friends on Facebook and claiming the results represented all America. That's pretty much what Kinsey did.

Kinsey was a pioneer. Everyone says it and it's true. He braved a wilderness most scientists were leery of and took the blows—and the rewards—that would have gone to any early entrant here. But he also stained the field, creating sensational, false impressions with methods that even a smart amateur would have avoided. As with Mead, many professionals still defend him. One book, coauthored by an anthropologist, puts Kinsey up on the plinth: "Kinsey was central in the creation of the scientific study of sex. He exemplified how such an emotionally charged subject could be studied with scientific rigor." The coauthor adds: "He advocated the sociological method of the survey of large populations with concern for representativeness and the 'statistical sense' without which one was 'no scientist.'"[8] College students reading books like this will think Kinsey was a careful practitioner of sampling.

At least one sexologist seems to acknowledge the errors—"Kinsey started this huge project before modern sampling methods had been devised"—but then amusingly cites the results as if they were valid.[9] Desire can warp perception. Scientists are vulnerable like other people, and therefore so is science itself. I believe Kinsey remains popular mainly as a hero of sexual liberation. He told America that pretty much everyone was cheating on his or her spouse, visiting sex workers, making homosexual contacts, and generally having a high old time. And if everyone was doing it, sexual deviants like myself (1975 Concurrent Sex Partner Champion of Greater Washington, D.C.) felt we weren't so deviant after all!

Start the Revolution with Me

When I was in college in the 1960s, the trenchant slogan "Make Love, Not War!" was everywhere. The war in Vietnam had tarred an older generation, pot smoke hung in the air, the noun "counterculture" appeared, and a new sensibility seemed poised to reshape society. Bob Dylan sang "The Times They Are a-Changin'," and *Hair* brought the "Age of Aquarius" to Broadway. And almost overnight sex became safe and available. The Pill had swept the world, and other contraceptives were easy to get. Deadly scourges like syphilis now yielded to a shot. New social forces like feminism upended people's ideas of sex roles. Pornography appeared in the convenience stores, clinics offered legal abortion, and *Oh, Calcutta!* brought a nudie show to off-Broadway.

Suddenly, exhilaratingly, people felt free. The ethic spread that full sexual expression was healthy for all. And, as with most revolutions, momentum carried it beyond the mark. To some, like New Age psychiatrists Norman O. Brown and R. D. Laing, the road of intercourse led to the palace of wisdom. By unshackling our repressed desires, we would actualize ourselves. As psychiatrist Theodore Dalrymple observed: "These enthusiasts believed that something beautiful would emerge: a life in which human pettiness would melt away like snow in spring." Yet, as he adds, the sexual revolution "foundered on the rock of unacknowledged reality."[10] People still sought love, the committed one-to-one bond, a genetic need related to the importance of the family in raising children. Women were also more vulnerable to abuse than men, and the revolution led to an enormous upsurge in violence between the sexes. As feminist Erica Jong told the *Washington Post* in 2005: "We thought sexual freedom would bring world peace. We really thought that if people gave up their inhibitions, the world would change. We were wrong."

Gay Paradise Lost

For most people the sexual revolution simply spiced up life, although the spice could be heady. But for gays it changed the universe. Suddenly, they could live as who they were. Many underwent radical transformations, going from isolation and shame to social acceptance and pride in their identity. Gay neighborhoods sprang up, like the Castro in San Francisco and West Hollywood in Los Angeles, where gay men could meet each other easily and openly. A world had emerged from underground. There was no going back.

But there would definitely be adaptation. Man2Man Alliance was formed by gay activists who had grown weary—then increasingly frustrated and angry—over the deaths of their friends, lovers, and life partners and the nonresponse (or response that made no public health sense) of the gay AIDS service organizations (ASOs) that had come to speak for *all* men who have sex with men (MSMs), allowing no other opinions to be heard. Here is a brief history of how that came about, from one of the silenced groups. Man2Man Alliance describes a three-stage movement in gay rights from tolerance toward rigidity. First came the mainstream era (c. 1950–1980), during which gay men sought to end discrimination, rioted in response to perceived police harassment at a now-famous spot in New York called Stonewall, and organized gay men and lesbians nationwide, yet they still honored the range of behaviors and values among themselves. However, the early idealism was "subverted and ultimately destroyed by economic, cultural, and biological forces which no Gay Liberationist anticipated." In the 1970s entrepreneurs arrived and spawned the proliferation of bathhouses, dark rooms, backroom bars, and other sex opportunity sites. Here, among a segment of gays, a fantastic promiscuity burst out. These men had hundreds of partners a year. The bathhouses hosted semipublic orgies every night, the most extravagant and extended parties in the annals of sex history. I worked on the Houston mayoral campaign in 1980 and because our (Hispanic) candidate asked me to help bring out the gay vote, a coworker and I went to a few bathhouses, where I glimpsed the activities firsthand. The reports were not exaggerated.

Then AIDS appeared, and suddenly each of these encounters carried the chance of annihilation. Indeed, given the early high-risk window, the newly infected could easily spread HIV to a variety of strangers in the bathhouse, who would then do the same, and so on. AIDS reached the West soon after the elections of Ronald Reagan in the United States and Margaret Thatcher in the United Kingdom, and coincided with the rise of Christian evangelism on TV and radio. Partly as a result, there was apathy at the top and a backlash from the right. Some solutions were pitiless: We should lock AIDS victims in quarantine camps. We should tattoo them, as William F. Buckley suggested. We should recriminalize homosexuality itself. "You have to remember that was the era when Jesse Helms and others were saying that gay people got what they deserved, and that the government shouldn't spend any money to help them," said David Evans, an HIV treatment advocate who writes about prevention. "There was a time when people thought, 'Oh my god, they're going to put us in camps.'"[11]

So the second stage in gay rights was reaction. Imagine you were a gay man back then. Your friends were dying, you were hearing it was your fault, and few in government seemed to care. Gay men *did* care about AIDS, passionately, and they became the first responders to the threat, along with contraceptive professionals like myself and the condom companies that sensed a market surge. Activists formed AIDS service organizations (ASOs)—including New York City's Gay Men's Health Crisis (GMHC), the San Francisco AIDS Foundation, and Shanti—and claimed that they alone cared about AIDS (when few others did, in fact). They understood it, these men claimed, and they knew how to fight it. Indeed, gay men were "instant experts" who presented themselves to USAID, the UN, WHO, and the other organizations that forged the global response to AIDS.

And in the third stage the ASOs helped codify the resistance into dogma. They drafted what they first called "safe sex" and later "safer sex" guidelines, based on condoms. Yet most early ASO members were the very people with the most at stake in keeping the party going. They were gay men who had acquired HIV through anal sex, and who identified so ardently with promiscuous anal sex that they felt all gay men should as well. Indeed, without AIDS, the Man2Man Alliance says, "it's likely that the pronounced predominance of anal promiscuity among gay men, which began around 1975, would have passed."[12] Instead, gays felt they had to present an army-like front to an attacking world.

The ASOs gained further credibility in the late 1980s, when incidence among U.S. gay men seemed to drop off. These organizations had us believe that gays had discovered how to achieve high levels of condom use—and thus, by implication, the saturnalia could continue. However, the decline almost certainly stemmed from die-off, as the greatest risk takers perished, and secondarily—as in Amsterdam—from a shift away from hazardous behavior, because of fear. Yet the notion that condoms could stop AIDS was now becoming orthodox belief. These activists still faced a fundamental challenge: How could they make mainstream society care? The answer: convince average people that they could get HIV too. Appeal to fear. Thus smart, effective activists worked to "de-gay" AIDS, to make it seem a universal threat.

At first many gays and straights working in AIDS genuinely did expect a heterosexual epidemic. But the tactic persisted long after evidence against one appeared. The tactic was stunningly successful, to the point that an unprecedented cash flow into AIDS has shifted global health funding away from child survival, clean water, environmental sanitation, and nearly every other area of public health, even in countries with HIV rates well below 1 percent, like India, which could use the money to save far more lives. As UN epidemiologist Elizabeth Pisani has described it: "HIV has changed the landscape of public health. It wasn't doctors who kick-started the response to this infectious disease, it was gay men. With a flair for dramatic presentation and an inside knowledge of what makes the communications industry tick, they battered down the doors of the medical establishment, assaulted the pharmaceutical industry, took the press by storm. They gave AIDS a political face. They were the production team that made AIDS different from the competing acts, that got AIDS started on its journey up the international development hit parade."[13]

So it's no wonder that gays have a sense of ownership about AIDS. They not only lost many thousands of friends and lovers to it, but they built a politically potent response to it against daunting obstacles. Indeed, gay AIDS experts and leadership became so entrenched that even the Bush administration appointed gay men to such posts as AIDS czar and second director of PEPFAR (the AIDS relief program begun in 2003). Although this response should humble the nongay outsider, the fact remains that 66 percent of all

HIV infections and 75 percent of all AIDS deaths occur in *Africa*, the great majority among heterosexuals. Tragically, the early gay line was correct for parts of Africa: AIDS is a heterosexual disease, statistically, and anyone can get it.

A Blame Game without Rules

One critic of liberal Big Brotherism has noted: "In order for victim groups to be worthy of (our) compassion, they must be entirely free of blame or responsibility for their misfortunes."[14] I hope this heartless remark is simply overstatement, and the writer would actually help, say, a cyclist who had negligently fallen from her bike. But those who developed and control the global response to AIDS are not inclined to blame the victim in any way. Fall off the bike and it's never your fault. Blame has been basic to this dynamic. Unlike almost any other health issue, victims here received a hot torrent of censure for the explosion of a disease. But in addition to punitive "solutions" like tattoos and camps, more moderate conservatives insisted that gays should cease being gay. They should just change their behavior. So the conservative message became one of *abstinence*. To gays, this response seemed oppressive, to say the least. They couldn't change their nature and didn't want to; "abstinence" seemed to mean a return to the closet from which they had so recently escaped. Hence the word "abstinence" developed an emotional charge.

At the same time some gays accepted no blame. Early on, gay author Randy Shilts wrote: "The politically correct line, emerging from a handful of 'AIDS activists,' maintained that talking about the gay community's prodigious promiscuity was part of a 'blame-the-victim mentality.'"[15] Indeed, some gay men engaged in sex acts they realized could kill their partners. Typhoid Mary didn't know her status, but these people did. Shilts tracked down dozens of stories of individual gays, as well as activists and bathhouse owners, who put their own sexual, political, and financial gratification over the lives of their gay brethren. The most notorious of these was "Patient Zero," the Canadian airline flight attendant Gaetan Dugas, whom scientists believe bears more responsibility for spreading AIDS in this country than anyone else. Forty of the first 248 cases of AIDS in the United States can be traced back to him, the first cases in New York and Los Angeles were linked to him, and as early as 1982, 11 AIDS cases arose from a single partner of Dugas.

AIDS researchers and gay activists identified Dugas while he was still alive. (He died in 1984.) Selma Dritz, a San Francisco public-health official, recalled a conversation with him in 1982. She asked him to stop deliberately infecting other people, and he responded: "It's my right to do what I want to do with my own body." Rapists could make the same claim, but even they don't go this far. Dugas had a receptive audience among some gays, who believed that an HIV-positive person had no duty to tell a potential sex partner of his illness. Lust came first and collateral damage was, well, sad. Now, I lost one of my best friends from college (Howard, who in those days was struggling with his sexual identity) to the excesses of 1970s San Francisco, including bathhouses. Someone like Dugas may have ended his life.

Yet the antigay label got pasted on critics of casual sex. Why was it antigay to want to stop gay deaths? Because conservatives, seen as antigay, were also against promiscuity. If the bad guys opposed it, all opponents were bad guys. That is, if penguins are birds and parakeets are birds, penguins are parakeets. For many, promiscuity was fun, a part of the gay lifestyle. Oppose the gay lifestyle and you must be antigay. However, because most gays live in ongoing relationships, *stability* is the real gay lifestyle. If this argument had any force, encouraging sexual freedom would be against the gay lifestyle and hence antigay. This tolerance of sexual homicide is still with us. For instance, on April 22, 2005, the gay student-activist Jonathan Perry gave the plenary speech at the Harvard AIDS Summit. Before he began, the student organizers presented him with a humanitarian award. During the applause some of Perry's friends rose to their feet, and because sitting quickly seems a snub in these situations, the remaining several hundred of us soon also stood.

Except we didn't know what the guy was going to say. Since Perry had become HIV-infected, he had spoken to numerous groups and appeared on *The Oprah Winfrey Show*, but his main activity seemed to be seeking men through the Internet for anonymous sex. He has "unprotected" anal intercourse, he said, and he doesn't tell his receptive partners he is HIV-positive. He related this story like a standup comedian, joking about his behavior for fifteen minutes. At one point he quipped, "Hey, if *you* don't care enough about your health to ask me about my HIV status, why should *I* tell you?" There was nervous laughter. No one revoked his humanitarian award or even questioned his behavior.

Why not? The jails are full of less dangerous people. One reason is a key weapon in the blame game: the charge of stigma. Anyone who enters AIDS World quickly hears the word. Certainly gays, prostitutes, and injecting drug users have suffered terribly from stigma. It has gone on for centuries, it continues, and it is disgusting and highly damaging. Yet many gays turned around and abused the word "stigma" itself, usually to help thwart funding for behavior change. This is similar to the reality that sometimes charges of racism discourage open discussion about African dictators. This term "stigma" deserves inspection. It is a powerful moral force, a toxic halo around individuals that deters others from imitating and even associating with them. For instance, most people stigmatize neo-Nazis, al-Qaeda members, serial killers, and child molesters. These are extremes, but the wish to avoid stigma keeps people behaving better. Stigma clearly has a purpose, which is why it evolved.

Epidemiologists Danel Reidpath and Kit Yee Chan have observed that stigma can serve an important health function.[16] Although the price is always some individual suffering, they note, stigma can benefit the population as a whole. The coauthors cite antismoking laws, which marginalize certain people but improve overall health and mortality rates. Because these laws encourage nonsmoking, they save many people from lung cancer, emphysema, and other harms much worse than stigma. Similarly, stigmas against drunk driving have reduced injuries and deaths. Thus as a negative incentive, stigma can keep us away from dangerous behavior. So stigma isn't necessarily wrong in itself. It can be immensely helpful. We simply have to aim it in the right direction. Yet in AIDS World we are conditioned to think that all stigma is bad, and we condemn it reflexively and immediately.

Even minor complaints can earn retorts of "stigmatizing," and of course "homophobic," "reactionary," and other slurs tend to accompany stigma. In other words, AIDS World tries to stigmatize its skeptics. At least, that's the sense one gets from hearing the repeated accusations. You can't have it both ways, though, and you especially can't condemn stigma if you're using it yourself. This blurring of moral focus has been tragic, because stigma can be a potent ally in fighting HIV. Although the price would be hurt feelings to the promiscuous, the gain would be countless lives saved. We saw it happen in Uganda. Despite this boon, however, too many people refuse to tolerate any price at all. So in AIDS World, we've stigmatized those who recommended sexual caution, and the price has been hurt feelings too, plus countless preventable deaths.

Bundling: First, Cure Poverty

AIDS is a viral disease. Certain sexual habits help it spread, and it's critical to modify them. Yet for years we have heard assertions that we can cut HIV infections by reducing poverty, racism, "classism," and other "isms." AIDS workers have hitched strategies like condoms to these glowing causes. It's called bundling. Bundling is understandable, to some extent. People who regularly work with high-risk, marginalized individuals deal with them on sensitive issues, and so must gain their trust and develop sympathy for them. Interventionists therefore easily get swept up into larger issues. Bundling also juiced the movement, making people feel satisfaction and camaraderie in fighting sexism, bigotry, hatred, capitalism, and Republican politics. Listen to Stephen Lewis, the UN secretary general's special envoy for HIV/AIDS in Africa, speaking about African nations in 2004:

> Where are the laws that descend with draconian force on those who are guilty of rape and sexual violence? Where are the laws that deal with rape within marriage? Where are the laws in every country that enshrine property and inheritance for women? Where are the new laws that protect women from stigma and discrimination? Where are the laws that raise the age of marriage? Where are the laws that abolish school fees, so that children orphaned by AIDS, with due emphasis on girls, can go to school? Where are the laws, or the regulatory apparatus, which guarantee that young women and girls, HIV positive, will have access to treatment in numbers that reflect the female prevalence rates? Where are the laws that guarantee equality before the law for women in all matters economic and social?
>
> In short, where are the laws which move decisively towards gender equality? No one disputes that there are profound changes in attitude and behavior required. But that can take generations, and in the meantime, we're losing the women and girls of Africa. It's wildly past time for the political leadership to produce the legal framework which will give women a chance to resist the virus.

That's great stuff. You can feel the exciting tug, and see how human rights came to permeate our entire approach to AIDS prevention. Yet the result has been devastating. When people tie a strategy to an ethically charged purpose, evidence becomes less important. A subtle conflict of interest arises. People start promoting the strategy to gain moral credit, and they tend to stop citing its flaws, to avoid attacks. These attacks can be vicious. Indeed, the quickest way to kill criticism of condoms has been to suggest that religious belief, conservatism, bigotry, patriarchy, homophobia, or sexism has polluted the dissenter's thinking.

Bundling has been acid to policy. Once the pro-condom position became synonymous with these goals, it became hard to focus discussion on the facts. Being anticondom was therefore seen as being anti–human rights. Bundling claims should have scared the wits out of AIDS workers. Imagine if we have to remedy poverty or gender inequality before we can prevent AIDS. If we have to make Kampala look like Denver, or even Buenos Aires, it's hard to guess how many more millions will die. We'll see why these claims not only didn't scare many AIDS activists, but actually appealed to them. At the same time, motivationally, it's impotent. How can a single person affect poverty or gender equality? Behavior change is like staying within the lines of a crosswalk; a person can do it alone and reduce her chance of harm. Changing gender equality is like changing citywide traffic patterns; no one can do it alone. Let's take an extreme case: suppose a very powerful corporate head gave women more and better jobs, raised their salaries, provided scholarships for them and their children, and worked to enhance their social status. The nationwide improvement in gender equality would still be slender and the reduction in HIV close to nil. How difficult is it to achieve gender equality? Look at Japan: even in this rich, sophisticated nation, gender inequality persists.

There is no credible evidence that gender inequality, poverty, discrimination, stigma, war and civil disturbances, racism, or homophobia actually drive HIV epidemics in *Africa*. Hence reducing these social ills will not reduce HIV infection rates, and the billions spent here are wasted, at least in terms of AIDS. And then there is the ultimate irony. Although bundling links strategies like condoms with electric-fence moral issues, the worst transgression in AIDS World is making moral judgments. The subtext must be: "*We* can moralize (because we're right), but *they* can't moralize (because *they* want to be the Sex Police)." Yet Africa challenges our assumptions. Its residents do make moral judgments about sexual behavior, and those are the people we have to work with and help. We can't turn them into us first.

. Bundling remains very much alive. When I was in Botswana in November 2007, the *Botswana Gazette* ran a prominent piece pushing politics, drugs, testing, and latex in the usual language of human rights. It said that more than thirty leading AIDS organizations had issued "an unprecedented joint declaration on the need to put legal and human rights protections at the center of HIV efforts." The document itself, written by the Open Society Institute, stated: "Human rights approaches to HIV are not abstract, but real, practical, and cost-effective. Countries that have placed human rights at the center of their AIDS responses have seen epidemics averted or slowed."[17] The declaration provided no traceable examples and it couldn't have in Africa. Similarly, a 2009 report from two Washington, D.C., NGOs concluded: "Responding to gender inequality is especially crucial for effective prevention, which will be key to limiting future costs." Such statements have pulled AIDS policy onto the rocks. Yet gender equality is crucial for reproductive health and so many other health issues, so it is understandable how this emphasis evolved, and of course I support it for these and a host of other good reasons.

Moral War: The Polarization

Bundling has increased the political friction. In his 1991 autobiography former U.S. Surgeon General C. Everett Koop addressed the issue early in the U.S. epidemic: "Unfortunately, most gay activists combined the otherwise separate issues of homosexual health and politics [such as access to jobs and housing]. They then placed this single package of grievances before the general public for redress." The upshot was more politicization than sympathy. "As a result,"

wrote Koop, "the first public health priority—to stop further transmission of the AIDS virus—became needlessly mired in the sexual
politics of the early eighties. We lost a great deal of time because of
this, and I suspect we lost some lives as well."[18] Indeed, AIDS has
become the most politicized disease in the annals of public health.
You don't see an us-versus-them mentality in cancer prevention, for
instance. But with AIDS some on the right have attacked condom
distribution in the same breath as broader contraception and progressive social programs. And some liberals have scoffed at behavior
change as part of a conservative agenda to "take back America."

Both sides have had trouble admitting the other might be even
partly right. Many Western experts, often with backgrounds in AIDS
activism and contraception, tend to be suspicious of religious organizations. There is a long history of antagonism between family-
planning organizations and certain religious groups, notably the
Roman Catholic Church. Indeed, before the Pill, condoms were the
main technological method of birth control, and liberals supported
their use while religious conservatives opposed it. These battle lines
descended down to the utterly different realm of African AIDS
prevention, and the old war continued on bizarrely inappropriate
grounds. Some of my family-planning colleagues still fear that any
criticism of condoms is an insidious wedge, evidence of a surrep-
titious project to ban funding for all contraception and block the
advance of women's rights.

The conflict reflects deeper values as well. Liberals tend to say,
"People are victims of social conditions, so don't expect fundamental
behavior change"; conservatives tend to say, "People are *more* than
that, so *do* expect fundamental behavior change." But because liberals ran the program, fidelity became an orphan. I recently discussed
these matters with my colleague the "comprehensive sex education"
guru Doug Kirby, and he commented that both sides in these debates
can and do abuse science, or at least cherry-pick the evidence that
supports their own view. He's right, of course. But I told him it was

beside the point. Only one side controls the billions of dollars that go to AIDS, so that side needs most correction.

Actually, I am not sure what "liberal" and "conservative" mean in AIDS World. To me, conservatives are the ones who defend a multi-billion dollar cartel from low-cost, sustainable, evidence-based solutions that work. Liberals are the ones who free the Third World from dependence on the West and respect the principles of public health.

Anthropology Enters the Maze

Anthropologists might have minimized ideology in Africa, because these Western scholars ought to know conditions on the ground. A key reason they didn't lies in the decline of anthropology itself. The field had once been a model of empiricism, but it has turned into a jousting ground of pet theories. I first encountered an early postmodern, activist researcher like this back in 1971, in the Amazon forest, where we were both working. I was surprised to discover he had not studied the basic literature on the area—neither geographical, topical, or theoretical. Nothing. It was all "honky hegemonic bullshit" He was not bothering to write field notes either. Yet this researcher was supposedly studying for his Ph.D. at a prestigious university. How would he pass his written exams, and what would he write his dissertation about?

Many of these new sub- or allied disciplines—social construction theory, postmodernism, sexology, erotics, queer theory, identity politics, lavender linguistics, gay and lesbian studies, deconstruction, feminist anthropology, and more—arose in, from, or in concordance with my own field of anthropology in the early 1980s. They gained sustenance from the global attention and the dollars that started flowing toward HIV/AIDS, first in a stream and then in a broad river. Some of these disciplines are hard to reconcile with the science of anthropology, not to mention epidemiology. For example, queer theory must restrict its analytic focus to discourse, rather than say, ethnography, making it "epistemologically incommensurable" with sociology or anthropology, according to critics like Adam Green. But they are not hard to reconcile with political activism. As one partisan noted, AIDS activists support "the pressing recognition that discourse is not a separate or second-order 'reality.'" But of course discourse isn't reality. It's an abstracted interpretation of a representation (ethnographic reports) of a representation (mental image) of reality. As abstractions are wont to do, it can lose touch with the world.

An anthology editor once asked me for a book chapter. Tongue-in-cheek, I told him that I had started working on one called "Pan-semiologism and Foreskins: A Hermeneutical and Sequential Analysis, Posing a Neo-Nonconstructivistic Approach to Epistemo-logical Rupture, While De-Emphasizing Representational Semiotic and Discursive Verificationals." I added that I had fallen into the Solipsist Trap and would be unable to finish the piece. Social construction theory itself emphasizes environmental factors, as opposed to the biological, in determining our sexual identity and behavior. Although the environment certainly plays a key role, overemphasis on it can breed highly misleading notions. Indeed, advocates of erotics, queer theory, feminist anthropology, and the like all argue that outlying sexual behaviors are relatively free from biology—while, in the AIDS context, claiming we can't change them. They exult in demonstrating that sexual behavior is far more varied than anthropologists ever considered, and see themselves on a mission to show how common and universal same-sex erotics and transgendered and intersexual behaviors are.

However, it was ethnography—fieldwork in non-Western cultures (later to become "cultures markedly different from one's own")—that once distinguished anthropology from nearly all other disciplines. Admittedly, it has grown harder to get funding and especially permission from postindependence Third World governments to do fieldwork in exotic cultures, to poke around among exploited groups and maybe take up their cause and make trouble for repressive regimes. But if no one had ever gone out into the field, we would have ignorance—that is, a marketplace of vague theories assembled from shreds of evidence.

Pillars of AIDS Ideology

Although it has myriad definitions, "ideology" is usually a rigid set of assumptions for guiding action. It typically exalts one value (such as freedom) with disregard for the reasons that make it a value. Ideologies almost always imply moral superiority—we're better than you—and that's why they so often appear in ethics-laden fields like politics. There, as in the *Divine Comedy*, delightful rewards await the orthodox and ghastly pains the dissenters. As Aldous Huxley wrote: "To be able to destroy with good conscience, to be able to behave badly and call your bad behavior 'righteous indignation'—this is the height of psychological luxury, the most delicious of moral treats." Ideologies also warp our view of the relevant evidence, making us ignore contradictory facts yet highlight congruent ones. People need not be aware of the process. In fact, they may not even realize they have an ideology, because it is a framework rather than a concept that one can easily hold in the mind, turn this way and that, and scrutinize. That makes ideologies more dangerous, for good people can follow them into bad places. Indeed, almost everyone mentioned in this book believes that he or she is saving lives.

AIDS ideology has three main pillars, each of which is discussed in detail below.

SEXUAL FREEDOM

The core belief here is that each person has the inalienable right to choose his or her sexual behavior and express it freely, without inhibiting judgments or censure from society. Throughout the first quarter century of AIDS prevention, this value has trumped essentially all other concerns, even health and life. The message has been, *Do it, and we'll help you do it safely.* An ideology of sexual freedom demands a technology that allows—perhaps encourages—unrestrained sex even in the era of HIV, even in ravaged Africa. Thus we see emphasis on using condoms, getting tested, and treating STDs, along with invitations to become advocates for sexual freedom and gay rights.

"Sex-positive" is the laurel bestowed on approaches that encourage sexual liberation. Condoms are therefore sex-positive because they don't limit sex. This term narcotizes serious thinking. It doesn't follow that, if sex is positive, all sex is positive. One might just as well say that food is positive, so overeating is "food-positive." Fishing is positive, so depleting the cod population is "fishing-positive." Energy is positive, so dropping an H-bomb is "energy-positive." Exalt one feature and ignore the rest, and the result can be disaster. But that's how ideology blinds people. Hence we saw precious few messages to reduce partners in the face of the epidemic. We saw few messages to not commit rape or seduce minors. We saw surprisingly few messages to avoid prostitutes, because, we heard, such advice might stigmatize sex workers, or at least make them feel less good about themselves.

An ideology of freedom is a special, highly intriguing case. It is what it reviles: a cage. This odd prison is surprisingly common. French revolutionary Robespierre praised "the despotism of liberty." In twentieth-century classical music freedom-seeking composers wrote extreme, often unpleasant works, partly because of attacks if they turned "conventional"—that is, if they exercised their freedom. And as gay philosopher Michel Foucault noted, "sexual liberation" was ultimately one more narrow role. Liberty is precious, yet ideology can constrict it in the name of liberty itself.

Pansexualism is a logical extension of sexual liberation. It is the belief that all consenting adult sex is good, and the more the better. Anything that gets in the way of more sex, or the fullest expression of the sexual impulse, is reprehensible. Pansexualism demands, for example, that a second-rate contraceptive be elevated to "the best weapon we have against AIDS," and not just for Africans but for gay men and indeed everyone, everywhere. As the gay activist group Man2Man Alliance depicts pansexualism, society shouldn't try to discourage any kind of sex act, "even if there's a high risk of disease." Instead, society has the obligation "to provide both education and the means which will enable individuals to do almost anything they please sexually with reduced risk of disease transmission. Which is the reason that condom campaigns are such a prominent feature of pansexualist public policy."[19]

This is AIDS prevention ideology in a nutshell. I am a Believer myself to some extent, but True Believers will go to any length to defend sexual freedom, or what the Marquis de Sade would have called *libertinage*. Thus, at a 2009 Harvard Law School debate on legalizing prostitution, a civil libertarian maintained that sexual intercourse with dogs or horses is fine as long as it's "consensual." And how would we know? According to Dr. Elizabeth Wood, we check to see if the dog is wagging its tail and the horse does not have its ears back. At least animal sex may be relatively safe (beyond a few swift kicks and the odd zoonotic disease). As gay liberation-ist Bill Weintraub, a leading critic of anal sex, recently observed, the "gay male community has an uncanny knack for latching onto practices which are dangerous, romanticizing them, exalting them into articles of faith, and then brutally attacking anyone who questions them. Anal (penetration), fisting, rimming, docking—just for starters."[20] Fisting, for instance, grossly distends tissue and causes membrane tears. Australian researchers have reported that some gay men are using crystal meth and erectile dysfunction medicines like Viagra for marathon sex. These artificially prolonged bouts can rupture condoms, bloody the penis or anus, and open easy avenues for the virus. Yet, as another commentator has noted: "As gay men have reaffirmed their gay identity by sexual expression, recommendations to change sexual behavior may be seen as oppressive. For many, safer sex has been equated with boring, unsatisfying sex."[21]

Of course, the same argument holds for reckless driving: if you find it exciting and fun, the laws against it are oppressive.

At the same time, pansexualism has led naturally to the bizarre blame-the-victim mentality noted earlier with the example of the HIV-positive student-activist Jonathan Perry. When he criticizes the men he infects, one might reasonably say he is blaming the victim. Yet those who question Perry's behavior get accused of blaming the victim (Perry himself). The fault lies not with the joyrider, but with the person who left the car unlocked. Pansexualism puts glands above life. So it is especially disturbing to hear these assertions from activists who also claim we must spend more and more money every year to fight AIDS. It is like hearing speeders urge more funds for hospitals to house people they've run over.

HARM REDUCTION

The second pillar in AIDS ideology is harm reduction. Can we change basic human behavior? The assumption that we can't is the key force behind the strategies of harm reduction—condoms, testing, any approach that leaves risky behavior unhampered. So instead of changing behavior we must try to mute its consequences. We won't build million-dollar levees, so we need billion-dollar pumps and water brigades. Harm reduction is a relatively recent idea. The term came into use only in about 1988, right in time for the AIDS pandemic and just as the programs in Amsterdam and Uganda were proving a better way—changing behavior. We can understand *harm reduction* better by contrasting it with *harm elimination*, in every sector where AIDS is a problem.

- In Africa the hazard is multiple ongoing partners, which creates sexual networks. *Harm reduction:* condoms, testing, and anti-retrovirals (ARVs). *Harm elimination:* fidelity and delay of debut.
- Among gays, the hazard is promiscuity and anal sex. *Harm reduction:* condoms, testing, and ARVs. *Harm elimination:* fidelity and avoidance of anal sex.

- Among prostitutes, the hazard is promiscuity. *Harm reduction:* condoms, testing, and ARVs. *Harm elimination:* changed employment, if possible.
- Among injecting drug users (IDUs), the hazard is dirty needles, high risk of HIV (as well as hepatitis B and C), and pressure into such lifestyle choices as crime and prostitution. *Harm reduction:* clean needle programs, smoking instead of injecting, and methadone substitution. *Harm elimination:* recovery, ending drug use.

Let me talk a moment about addiction, where you might think behavior change would be least effective, because the problem is *compulsive* behavior, driven by obsessive thinking. First, don't get me wrong: for those who cannot or will not give up heroin, harm reduction is certainly better than nothing. Methadone is more addictive than heroin, yet using it is infinitely less risky than mainlining a substance alleged to be heroin, brought off the streets, of unknown strength or purity that might be rat poison. It can also be a first step toward ending the risk behavior altogether. My problem is that we *only* do harm reduction for IDU epidemics, just as until very recently we have *only* promoted risk reduction for sexually transmitted epidemics. Although a single clean needle is virtually 100 percent safe, as is a correct methadone dose, the programs themselves are only modestly effective, and the addiction continues.

An often-repeated argument for harm reduction goes like this: If we cannot end, say, the drug habit for everyone, why try to end it for anyone? Similarly, in Africa we hear that fidelity won't protect every faithful wife, so it's pointless to promote fidelity at all. This claim is absurd on its face, but it is staggering to hear it from a proponent of harm reduction, someone who admits her *own* program won't protect everyone. Yet some very competent people have brought forth this rationale.

Here is a strange fact: the great majority of drug (and alcohol) treatment facilities in America and many other countries aim at complete abstinence from all mood-altering substances. True, abstinence-oriented programs like Alcoholics Anonymous don't work for everyone. But this approach has been shown to succeed better than any other, and there are a great many thousands of former heroin addicts in America alone. Even a move from needles to smoking would save great numbers of lives, because the virus can't travel in vapor. So harm elimination constitutes "best practice" for at least the Unites States. Yet this is not the approach we export to meet the challenge of HIV transmission among IDUs—that would be harm reduction, with clean needle and methadone programs. It's almost as if we hold people in the less-developed world to a lower standard. We assume they can't control themselves, so we hand them the second best.

A kind of vicious circle is at work here. Belief in harm reduction has put AIDS partly in the hands of health economists and medical professionals. They are far more comfortable with condoms, drugs, and medical devices than with the complexities of sexual or addictive behaviors—especially when powerful groups of AIDS activists were saying, in effect, don't touch either. These experts have perpetuated the approach.

CULTURAL RELATIVISM

The third pillar in AIDS ideology is cultural relativism. Are moral standards inherent and universal, or does the culture shape them? Cultural relativism is the belief that there are no absolute standards of right and wrong, or good and bad, or anything else. Cultural relativism originates from anthropology, where it has at least two widely shared meanings. The first is strictly practical. When I worked with the Matawai, I suspended my own moral judgments about their behavior. (It was easy, because they were *very* moral. For example, there had been only one homicide in the century before my visit.) I sought a modicum of understanding or empathy with their rules, norms, and proclivities. This approach is essential, for otherwise it's hard to convey findings objectively, in a way that yields insight to others. Moral judgments degrade observation itself. If a person thinks a practice is "bad," he tends to see it less clearly. Overall, the values of the observer upstage the evidence.

The second meaning of cultural relativism is intrinsic. There really are no absolute standards, and the culture of other people is no less than our own. The mores of the gay culture, for instance, are thus beyond criticism, because any ethical judgment merely imposes our own culture-bound standards on them. Morals are socially constructed, like table manners. A practice is wrong because it isn't ours. Of course, questions arise at once: Do we nod approvingly as Nazi guards haul bodies to the crematoria, unwilling to impose our culture-bound standards on them? Do we say the Aztec mass sacrifices were moral because the killings were "moral to them"? Or, in a more recent example, do we side with those who defended Cuba's former national policy of sending HIV-positive Cubans to quarantine villages? If so, was that approach "moral" up until the minute Cuba's leaders decided to end it? Can dictators determine ethics?

Evolutionary psychologists have persuasively described the origin of morals among early humans on the African savanna over the past two million years. Ethics arose because they enhance cooperation, which in turn helps keep people alive. So in generation after generation, ancient folks with genes for cooperation left behind more descendants, and therefore more genes for cooperation. Eventually they spread to everyone. Hence we have strong moral emotions like revenge and guilt, and an understanding of fundamentally good and bad behavior across cultures. Nature interacts with nurture, of course, so the specifics vary, but morals are not just table etiquette.

These three components—sexual freedom, harm reduction, and cultural relativism—fed into a vigorous ideology, and as a result, we have always treated AIDS differently from other diseases, the phenomenon called "AIDS exceptionalism." As the author of a 2006 article observed, the concept "consists of significant deviations from what otherwise would be standard public health practice in the areas of infection control, surveillance, partner notification, and testing."[22] We don't require HIV testing or notifying partners that they are at risk of a fatal disease. We don't usually recommend sexual behavior change—or even discuss it. We ignore Uganda.

AIDS was characterized as an "emergency" rather than as a preventable disease, even by the Bush administration, which allocated an unprecedented fifteen billion dollars to the president's emergency fund for AIDS relief (PEPFAR). It put most of that money into treatment with expensive drugs, itself a violation of the public-health principle that you prevent a disease first rather than trying to rein in its consequences later. We have offered a variety of excuses for these anomalies. The authors cited above explained: "Public health leadership has had reservations about the adverse impact of AIDS exceptionalism, but has been complicit with it for many years out of respect for people infected with and affected by HIV and AIDS."[23]

Get it? "Public-health leadership" suspected this approach was killing large numbers of people but didn't act, out of respect for those already ill. And for those merely "affected by HIV." This is truly interesting stuff. No one shows this ghastly "respect" for victims of heart disease, thankfully, and public-health leadership could show the greatest respect for current sufferers by preventing their friends and lovers from getting sick. I suggest these leaders are in the harness and clip-clopping over bad ground, and their "respect" is really fear of the ideological lash.

Bringing the Ideology to Africa

Many of the first "experts" the West sent to Africa were gay men who had little or no experience outside U.S. cities like San Francisco and Los Angeles. These men meant very well, but one of the consequences was that many Africans could dismiss AIDS as not a threat to themselves. Homosexuality remains illegal and very hidden in much of sub-Saharan Africa. Many Africans, seeing openly gay men for the first time and simultaneously learning from AIDS experts about the "gay plague" in America, reasoned: "Well, that's not us. We don't do anal sex with men, so we can't get this new disease." I have heard people say—very much in private—that we might have lost ten or more years of AIDS prevention by sending gay men as our first emissaries against the new pandemic. Some of us realized this at the time, but none dared say it in public. Needless to say, such observations are ultra-sensitive, and it's almost impossible to raise the subject without being accused of homophobia. Such a charge could end a career in AIDS overnight. But ten years translates into millions of lost lives.

These AIDS ambassadors created a gay-friendly or at least "sex-positive" program for Africa. In the name of AIDS prevention, we have sought to defeat homophobia in Africa, to champion the rights of sexual minorities, and normalize or reduce the stigma from prostitution. And we have told ourselves that we are being sex-positive, that we're being "values-free," that we're being unbiased and nonjudgmental, that we're spreading freedom. Now, I might personally believe in this freedom. But the goal is stopping the spread of AIDS, and to do so we have promoted a Western ideology to relatively conservative, mostly rural and religious, agricultural peoples of Africa and elsewhere. When they resist, we pity them for their backwardness, their "failure to understand," when it is *we* who have failed to understand the cultures where we intervene.

We tell doctors, "First, do no harm," and we mean it. If a physician makes a foolish error and a single patient suffers, the doctor is liable for malpractice. He may have to pay the injured party a huge sum of money. Yet if public-health organizations make foolish errors again and again and again, and calamity ensues, there is no malpractice. There is no remedy at all. The dead have "failed to understand."

CHAPTER 7

Ins and Outs of the Castle

My colleague Rand Stoneburner, who estimated that fidelity could have saved millions in South Africa alone, had hit the same surprise glass walls I had. He'd speak and, as he recounted, the people in AIDS World would try "to come up with some explanation to dismiss the data, from blaming laboratory error to bringing up every imaginable bias." Stoneburner felt the world had gone mad. Yet the forces were quite earthly. Here's how he put it: "When I was finally able to get people to talk about [Uganda], they would ask me, 'What are the implications for this with respect to funding?'"[1]

We've seen the implications. Most of that funding isn't necessary. Uganda slashed AIDS on five million dollars a year. These people weren't afraid programs would cost *more*. They were afraid programs would cost *less*. All our money supports a mega-structure. Imagine you are an African in a village and occasionally you see people handing out condoms at the clinic and providing information on AIDS. You might sense a vast invisible castle above this clinic, where officials decide on strategies and from which money cascades down. But you would never see it. You'd be sensing AIDS World. Unlike that villager, we can take a look at it.

AIDS World is a potent alliance of wealthy-country elites who benefit from a cash-rich industry. It consists, roughly, of two tiers. At the top are the original donors. They include governments and multinationals like the World Bank and the United Nations, as well as such major, liberal-oriented foundations as Gates, Clinton, Soros, Ford, Hewlett, and Packard. Taxpayers fund the first tier (directly or indirectly), and consumers and investments the second tier. Below them we find the providers, the "coalition of the billing," which we can divide into the nonprofits (like CARE International and Save the Children) and the for-profit organizations (like Family Health International, Population Services International, and The Futures Group), to mention five organizations I have consulted for. As some names suggest, many of these organizations specialize in family planning and contraception, in part because the U.S. government and other major donors made birth control (a term we *never* use, even in jest) such a high funding priority before AIDS edged it to a distant second place. Staffers at this level tend to be advocates of gender equity, gay rights, and reproductive health and family planning as well as international development professionals. I myself share these views.

The Fountainhead: Original Donors

In 2008 a record $15.6 billion was available to fight AIDS in low- and middle-income countries (although UNAIDS complained that this sum was too low, by $6.5 billion). About half of it, $7.7 billion, came from donor governments, and the United States provided slightly more than half (51.3 percent) of that amount. The United Kingdom followed with about one-eighth (12.6 percent), and the Netherlands, France, and Germany each contributed about one-six- teenth (6 percent) each. Hence these five nations contributed more than 90 percent of the aid, and no other country accounted for more than 2 percent. Domestic governments supplied about $7.2 billion to efforts in their own countries, although in destitute nations this amount was typically small—in Uganda's case, for instance, 6 per- cent of the total for fighting AIDS.

In 2008 the total sum was 39 percent or $4.4 billion greater than in 2007. This inrush of cash seems to have caused disorientation and lost opportunities. According to a 2010 UNAIDS document, the rise in number of AIDS groups and workers in each country "often overwhelms national efforts" and results in "piecemeal actions against AIDS that are often duplicative and rarely sustainable." So source donors like USAID hear both that they need to give more and that their money is getting squandered. USAID is the agency that distributes U.S. government funding for African AIDS, and AIDS in many parts of the world. It hands out most U.S. foreign aid of all kinds, and in 2008 it dispensed about $3.9 billion to battle AIDS in all middle- and low-income nations. As the largest donor in AIDS, it wields vast power. I know from personal and professional experience that USAID/Uganda has long felt that fidelity and delay of sexual debut are unrealistic strategies. It has also favored sex-positive messages instead of fear appeals, political appointees during the Bush administration notwithstanding.

The first director of the USAID program AIDSCOM (1986–1993), Glen Margo, rejected fear as a motivator. "These campaigns may temporarily discourage sexual activity," he said, "but then there is a boomerang effect as people react against the scare tactics." Similarly, a volume on AIDSCOM criticized HIV fear appeals as crude attempts to "scare people into abstaining" from sex. Moreover, fear would fail: "Early scare campaigns seem to have little impact on people's actions." This extraordinary misperception was orthodoxy among American AIDS experts. For example, a 1990 Institute of Medicine report observed that AIDS prevention was still a new endeavor, a "beginning technology." Yet, it continued, "we know for example, that public responses to fear messages is [sic] not optimal. It results in short-term behavior change but no behavior change over the long run."[2] However, the report provided no evidence to support this claim.

In dismissing fear appeals, AIDSCOM itself relied on several eastern Caribbean health surveys that focused on condoms only. These researchers equated fear with "perceived severity"—that is, the perceived magnitude of harm: How bad is AIDS? More realistic measures would have been "perceived susceptibility" or "personal risk": What's my chance of getting HIV? Or, even more accurately, how frightening was the message: Did it scare me? In the American experts' view, people responded better to a "more lighthearted, upbeat approach." Hurricane Katrina is coming, but let's be "weather-positive." The goal was to promote a healthy, active sex life (whatever one's sexual orientation) through feel-good messages. One poster from the Dominican Republic showed a baseball player about to hit a ball out of a stadium with the caption: "It doesn't matter what play I'm making: I protect my bat!" Such a message falls flat on the ears of people who have not gone through the sexual revolution, but one article cited it as an example of a good AIDS prevention poster.

Similarly, an ad in Botswana showed a fourteen-year-old girl who smilingly tells us she had added flavor (and by implication, gifts and an allowance) to her life by entering into a sexual relationship with a man twice or more her age—and she could do it by using Lovers Plus condoms "every time," funded by the U.S. taxpayer. This ad encouraged the sugar-daddy phenomenon Uganda had outlawed as defilement. Botswana soon made the U.S. contractor pull the ad, but Africans only push back in rather extreme circumstances. Imagine running this ad in the United States, especially in a rural, Bible-belt area. Imagine people—especially but not only in such an area—learning that "we" are creating and running an ad like this, anywhere. It gets even wilder, though. In Trinidad and Tobago in 1989 an AIDS prevention pamphlet from WHO advised primary school kids: "Do not urinate in the mouths of your friends." Parents and teachers were outraged and protested at the local WHO office. This pamphlet had come from a San Francisco program and kept the original urolagnia fetish content. It had simply been "tailored" for Trinidad by inserting photos of black kids near palm trees.

A later USAID program was AIDSCAP (AIDS Control and Prevention), which Family Health International ran from 1991 to 1997.

It tested for HIV and alleviated STDs, and its guidelines for workers stressed use of condoms and seeking treatment for STDs. "It was considered too moralistic to stress abstinence and fidelity," recalled David Wilson, a USAID consultant in Zimbabwe. In fact, it was considered too moralistic even to mention them as options. Today the Uganda AIDS Commission is finally reconsidering fear appeals. Top national officials have urged their deployment, and the commission's director general, David Kihumuro Apuuli, recently stated: "We have to change the destiny of this country, even if it means putting back the drums of the 1980s that used to frighten people."[3] But the final decision remains unclear because, as we will see, Ugandans do not really get to make such decisions.

The Second-level Donors

In 2008 donors gave $5.7 billion to developing governments and $2.1 billion to agencies like the World Bank, UNAIDS, and the Global Fund to Fight AIDS, Tuberculosis, and Malaria (known simply as the Global Fund). The latter become donors themselves and play a key role, distributing money to providers on the ground. They supply the expertise and contacts governments lack, but they also add a layer of management and, as in corporations, they reduce transparency looking down. In 2008 they provided more than three-quarters of the international assistance for AIDS in more than seventy countries, and between half and three-quarters in another thirty countries.

The World Bank. Along with the International Monetary Fund (IMF), the Washington, D.C.–based World Bank is one of the great supra-national institutions of the global economy. Created in 1944, it has 185 member countries that funnel money to it and have powers similar to shareholders in a cooperative. The World Bank provides grants and technical expertise to poor nations (and loans to middle-income ones), supporting projects in areas across the development spectrum, including education, energy, agriculture, and health. In

2008 it gave Africa five billion dollars in loans and grants for all purposes. The World Bank was slow to rally against AIDS. From 1988 to 1999 it spent an average of fifteen million dollars per year to quell the disease in Africa. Its efforts picked up around the millennium, and in 2009 its Multi-Country HIV/AIDS Program (MAP) gave five hundred million dollars to local organizations and communities to battle AIDS.

The Global Fund. The Global Fund sprang up in January 2002 to broaden the worldwide funding stream for AIDS, tuberculosis, and malaria. Today, as a foundation incorporated in Switzerland, it obtains, manages, and hands out funds, and in 2008 it dispensed a total of $1.03 billion to 136 low- and middle-income countries. The fund says it provides "a quarter of all international financing for AIDS globally, two-thirds for tuberculosis and three-quarters for malaria." Although the United States has given the fund millions for malaria and tuberculosis, it has reserved most of its AIDS monies for PEPFAR. In 2009 the head of the Global Fund was one of those to attack Pope Benedict XVI for criticizing condom distribution. At the outset the fund asserted that it would focus with special care on accurate measuring and evaluation. Hence the embezzlement scandal that enveloped it in 2006—with tens of millions of dollars stolen, by local estimates, or about the cost of Uganda's entire early program—was especially embarrassing. Corruption is rife in much of Africa, but the Global Fund knew that, and the affair made some wonder how, if the fund couldn't keep track of disbursements, it could accurately gauge results.

UNAIDS. The most prominent AIDS-only intermediary is Geneva-based UNAIDS, the United Nations clearinghouse for AIDS information and outreach. It is primarily an organization for fundraising and advocacy, and it receives major donations from Western governments and foundations. It does no research. Describing UNAIDS when she joined in 1996, Elizabeth Pisani says that "we sat in our offices and talked passionately about hookers, johns, queens, fags, whores, rent boys, trannies, junkies and smack heads." Pisani admits that she and her colleagues spent a lot of time worrying who was most politically correct. For example, some frowned on her use of "subpopulation" for gay men and intravenous drug users, because "the term may cause distress to some stigmatized groups by suggesting they are somehow 'beneath' mainstream society." Clearly UNAIDS was not focused on the majority population in Africa, where the worst of the epidemic was taking lives.

UNAIDS has been called "the most trusted source of scientific information on the global epidemic," yet it violated that trust repeatedly. As the world would eventually learn, UNAIDS spread falsehoods as a matter of at least informal policy, assuring themselves it was for a good cause. Its erstwhile director, Peter Piot, is an esteemed scientist and a humane, dedicated individual, like so many others in this field, but ideology has narrowed his thinking. For instance, in the past few years he has switched from urging evidence-based AIDS prevention to evidence-*informed* prevention. It's the difference between "We will follow the evidence wherever it leads us" and "We will use the evidence we like." Obviously, this approach permitted bias in African AIDS prevention, where there was a desperate need for impartiality. We have seen the same mind-set in the Vietnam and Iraq wars: the selective evidence-informed decisions, the rejection of crucial facts, and the fiasco. We see this with every ideology.

How did Piot justify this declaration? As he said in a speech, "If we only go for evidence-based, it means we take a purely technocratic approach that does not include human values." So UNAIDS would put its view of values ahead of evidence. He had two choices: (1) a "purely technocratic" approach, *based on evidence*, that would save more lives; and (2) a values-influenced approach, *informed by evidence*, that would save fewer lives. I am still trying to figure out what values could justify letting Africans die. Of course, the terms were misleading too. The true technocratic approaches were those like condoms, which required technological manufacture and brought in technician-bureaucrats from abroad. Uganda used human nature and built on the understandings, institutions, and cultures—including Ugandan values—of affected communities.

It is hard not to speculate that UNAIDS is *using* AIDS, that it has made the disease the centerpiece of fear appeals to spur social reforms. That is, reform is the value it puts ahead of evidence and public health. At the same time UNAIDS has become fixated on raising money, on means rather than ends, and it has learned which approaches work best. Many organizations seek to improve poverty and gender equality, for instance, and the more they believe these goals jibe with AIDS prevention, the more they contribute. And so the money comes in, organizations spend it on sex-positive messages and enticements to use condoms, and the cemeteries keep filling.

Rubber Barons:
The Family-planning Organizations

Most of the AIDS prevention billions ultimately reach family-planning organizations—and promotion of contraceptives is their raison d'être. Yet ties to family planning, a health industry perhaps second only to HIV/AIDS in global funding levels, do not come baggage-free. There are obvious biases toward contraceptive solutions, or at least toward solutions based on commodities. The pro-condom bias is so oceanic it tends to goes unnoticed—or at least unmentioned. In published scientific research today, authors typically reveal their connections to an industry up-front in conflict-of-interest statements. For example, authors of a recent *Lancet* article on "generalized anxiety disorder" detail the bonds between themselves and more than a dozen drug companies as well as trusts, private foundations, and other journals and councils. They acknowledge accepting paid speaking engagements in industry-supported symposia at national and international meetings. Hence *Lancet* readers can judge whether these links taint the questions investigated, the findings, and the analysis. This is as it should be. But authors rarely mention their ties to family planning and AIDS organizations (and funding). These connections fall under every definition of "conflict of interest" one can think of, yet I am the only person I know of who has raised this issue. It deserves much wider discussion.

So do the larger scale abuses. For instance, PSI, one of the world's largest social-marketing companies, receives a hundred million dollars or more a year to sell condoms to Africans. A few years ago, perhaps wondering how to expand their market, PSI executives conducted a survey of Zambians and found that the main reason people didn't use condoms in last sex was trust of one's partner, at 42 percent. At the same time, few Zambians cited cost as a barrier to condom use. To understand the trust "problem" better, PSI conducted a follow-up, multi-country qualitative study. It found that the phenomenon was widespread. Youth in all nations examined "placed a high value on sexual fidelity and its role in trusted partnerships."[4] These findings in hand, PSI launched a campaign to make people *mistrust* their partners. The organization explained that husbands and wives could not really know if their spouses were cheating. And of course HIV had serious consequences. Hence less trust was healthy and spouses should use condoms more.

Unfortunately, mistrust in marriage doesn't lead to more condom use. It leads to violence against women and divorce. How did PSI executives get away with spending taxpayer dollars on such an enterprise? They gave it an Orwellian name—the Trusted Partner campaign—and promoted it as a defense of helpless women. They said they were out to stop philandering husbands who infect their wives by refusing to use condoms every time they have marital sex. The campaign undermined fidelity, marriage itself, and abstinence, and thus invited greater chance of HIV infection.

Indeed, the family planners and their allies have attacked marriage as "the most dangerous thing an African woman can do." UNAIDS propagated this falsehood and as recently as 2008, Stephen Lewis, former ambassador for UNAIDS, said in a Dan Rather interview: "It has been repeatedly pointed out that one of the riskiest propositions for a woman today in Africa is to be married."[5] In fact, however, married Africans are virtually *always* less likely to be infected than unmarried men and women of the same ages. The data could not be clearer: marriage is a relative haven. Studies have shown that African women are most likely to contract HIV in the period *before* marriage. But African women listening to this Western advice increased their chances of getting HIV.

Most African teens are not sexually active, unless they are already married, according to our best surveys. Fidelity and delay programs deal with such populations not currently at risk, but these silent majorities are of no interest to condom companies. Only the sexually active buy latex, so an ideology of sexual freedom does not hurt revenue. At the same time, contraceptive organizations will continue to steer the AIDS billions toward high-risk groups such as sex workers, gay men, and injecting drug users, thus directing it away from the real population at risk in Africa. The most ironic perk of promoting condoms for AIDS is that people feel virtuous for helping the needy and the outcast.

Big Pharma: Prevention versus Infection?

At the 1998 World AIDS Conference part of the official agenda was the "Cultural Programme and Useful Hints." It told attendees where to go for "backroom sex" in "hardcore" and "cruising" bars. No moralistic judgments here. In fact, the sex-positive message was, *Hey guys, we—Big Pharma, the sponsors of the world's largest scientific conference—are on your side!* These sponsors were mainly Merck (protease inhibitors), Bristol Myers Squibb (protease inhibitors), Glaxo-Wellcome (patent on AZT), Upjohn, Roche, Abbot Labs, and Dupont Pharma. At international AIDS conferences I've seen pamphlets printed by drug companies that tell men where to go locally for anonymous sex with other men. Big Pharma is hardly the biggest force in this arena, but it faces its own conflict of interest with AIDS. Having worked in contraceptive social marketing, I know that condoms cost only a couple of pennies to make. Nonetheless, profits are meager on condom sales, at least in developing countries. Drug companies would rather turn from selling condoms to far more profitable AIDS drugs or lifestyle enhancers like Viagra. In other words, and this is key: *they make less money by preventing HIV than treating it.*

Is it possible that the large pharmaceutical firms don't want behavior to change? I know some of these executives, and it is plain to me that, as family members and churchgoers, they want at-risk individuals to act safely. These are decent, caring people like most of us. But pharma companies are huge, complex organizations with many divisions, employees, and cross-currents, and less risk means less profit. Drug companies forged alliances early on with gay activist groups like ActUp, and actually funded them secretly to travel to conferences so they could demand more money for AIDS and "fast-tracking," namely swifter FDA approval, meaning less research for AIDS drugs. For instance, the FDA approved AZT to treat certain patients with AIDS on March 20, 1987, within just four months of receiving a new drug application from Burroughs Wellcome. Of course, fast-tracking means more profits. The firms also finance gay magazines like *Poz* and *Positive Nation*, which serve corporate interests by demanding lower standards for drug approval and more money for research. It has all meant bigger bottom lines for pharma companies.

Faith-based Organizations

Most Africans are highly religious, and faith-based organizations (FBOs) provide many of the health and education services and facilities in Africa, including those related to AIDS. As noted, the "Big Three" on the continent—Anglicans, Catholics, and Muslims—all helped control Uganda's epidemic early on. They have great sway in Africa, whether Western AIDS experts approve or not, and like the vast majority of Africans, they are very comfortable with anyone promoting fidelity and abstinence.

Indeed, I have always been struck by the extraordinary amount of AIDS prevention and care that FBOs provide around the world, usually with little funding. Muslim, Christian, Buddhist, Hindu, and Jewish organizations work hard to fight stigma, poverty, and other consequences of the disease, and contribute immensely to HIV prevention, support, and care of African families. The Catholic Church sponsors around 27 percent of all AIDS-related services worldwide, and in Africa alone the Church works in nearly a thousand hospitals, more than five thousand clinics, and eight hundred orphanages. A 2007 WHO study found that FBOs owned between 30 percent and 70 percent of the health infrastructure in Africa. Christian health centers provide about 40 percent of HIV care and treatment services in Lesotho and almost a third in Zambia, yet often there is poor coordination between them and public-health agencies. FBOs also help reduce stigma. In fact, a survey I published through USAID showed that fighting AIDS-related stigma is one of the main strengths and activities of FBOs working in Africa.[6]

That article proved to be the last of mine that USAID would publish, even though it had commissioned me to do two more studies. The story is telling. Late in the Clinton administration, I volunteered to write a USAID monograph on the role of FBOs in AIDS prevention, after the man originally commissioned became too sick to do it. I think USAID expected me to write a fluff piece along the lines of: "Everyone needs to be involved in fighting AIDS, FBOs are part of 'everyone,' ergo FBOs should be involved." Instead, I emphasized the advantage FBOs enjoy in promoting fidelity and abstinence in Africa. It took several years of struggle to get this monograph published by a USAID contractor. At least twice it was literally yanked from the publisher at the last moment, and not because of the contractor. In an e-mail to me and a dozen others, the AIDS activist at USAID in charge of liaison between the USAID Office of HIV/AIDS and the FBOs expressed his conviction that FBOs have no place in prevention, because all they do is "stigmatize and moralize." I finally brought enough political pressure to force its publication, but it emerged stripped of its cover and all photographs. It was the only monograph in the series to appear in cheap white paper with no pictures of any sort. FBOs remain underutilized. As recently as October 2009, Monsignor Robert Vitillo, the special adviser of Caritas Internationalis to the UN, said: "Government agencies often bypass faith-based organizations even though they're doing the bulk of the work."

What are my own religious beliefs? I would hardly bring the matter up if so many others hadn't made inappropriate assumptions. I have always presented myself as an agnostic to the press and to anyone else who asks. I don't want my findings about AIDS to be dismissed as the propaganda of a religious zealot. But the fact is, I have a hard time believing that the universe could have come about through random processes. I believe in a Prime Mover of it all and I've already mentioned my Episcopalian pedigree, yet I don't attend any church nor do I belong to any religious organization. I have recently become friends with an Iranian who happens to be a Zoroastrian (or Zarathustrian) and I find this religion rather appealing, especially because it lacks a clerical bureaucracy between Man and Maker.

But as an anthropologist and humanist, I do not upset myself over *other people's* religious beliefs or affiliations. Most Africans are highly religious, whether Christian or Muslim, and so religion matters very much to *them*. If we are truly trying to help Africans defeat AIDS or develop economically, it should matter not in the least whether Ted Green or anyone else from the helping side is religious or atheist. Faith-based organizations are very powerful in Africa. A rule of thumb might be "the poorer the country, the more important the role of FBOs." African FBOs own and operate a great many schools, clinics and hospitals, not to mention charities for the disabled, and they do a lot of other good works. If we have any sense at all, we work *with* religious organizations and not at cross-purposes with them. As a Ugandan colleague likes to say, we bypass them at our own peril. We *need* them to access the masses.

I have done a few evaluations of the projects of World Vision, a Christian organization. One was actually for a secular nonprofit scanning Mozambique for good examples of sustainable primary health care, and I concluded that World Vision had one of the best. Later, I evaluated a Balkan project it funded with its own money (that is, not the U.S. government's) aimed at assisting Muslim Gypsies who had been expelled from Kosovo and were living in Montenegro. At one point I asked a Gypsy leader what it was like to receive help from a Christian organization. He wanted to know what I was talking about. "Well, World Vision," I said. "You know, they're a Christian organization." He didn't know. He said the World Vision guy they dealt with was a Muslim from a Kosovo mountain tribe . . . and why was I asking? I told him that World Vision has been accused of seeking converts to Christianity while doing charitable aid work in various countries with U.S. government funds. This Gypsy leader exclaimed: "Who is telling these lies? Bring them to me, I will set them straight!" Other Gypsy leaders I spoke with felt the same.

I realized that these World Vision (or Catholic Relief Services, or Mennonite Central Committee, or many other) workers have something profoundly important in common with "target audiences" in Africa that people from secular organizations often lack: religion. It might infuriate AIDS activists to point this out, but there it is.

The Real World of Africa

In 2010 the United States overhauled its health-care insurance system to provide coverage for all. Such coverage everywhere else on earth has improved lifespan and quality of life, and the United States was alone among industrialized nations in not providing it.

Africa and most developing countries have a different system, called "out-of-pocket." Only the rich, the military, and some government workers have any insurance at all. So if you get sick, you pay the cost yourself. No money, no treatment. (The big exception has been AIDS programs, awash in poorly spent money.) Indeed, in most parts of Africa there is no medical service at all as Westerners know it. That's one reason why life expectancy in Zambia is thirty-five and in Mozambique it's thirty-two, and why rural Africans think Western visitors are much younger than they really are.

When Africans get sick, most consult traditional healers, and as a result, they share an African worldview in which sex is believed to be potentially dangerous. Both patient and healer understand a number of genitourinary symptoms as relating to "contamination" with "impure" sexual fluids (such as those from a promiscuous partner), the "shadow of death" (the taint of mortality widows carry until the purification ceremony), and menstrual blood. Extramarital sex can lead to an illness believed to come from "husband's protection" (*likhubalo* in Zulu and Swazi), a spell or potion the husband puts on (or in) the wife, so that if she has sex with another man, that man becomes seriously ill. These are some of the social control mechanisms, hidden from foreign AIDS experts, that still operate today. Many of these controls conflict with Western-promoted notions that sex is merely recreational and that guilt-free sex is a human right.

I made these observations and showed supporting evidence in a 1994 book about how indigenous healers understand STDs and AIDS. I discovered that throughout sub-Saharan Africa people attribute a great many illnesses and misfortunes to having sex with the wrong kind of partner. In Mozambique, for instance, healers tell clients to avoid or be wary of sex partners outside the home, especially prostitutes and soldiers. They are also guardians of traditional African ideas of morality and commonly say that neglect of tradition and violation of the moral code—especially sexual prohibitions—leads to a bevy of diseases. However, today's economic factors, population, and migration have weakened much of this regulation. In South Africa I interviewed a variety of traditional healers who agreed that morality in the past few generations had eroded, leading to increased sexual permissiveness. Some healers have blamed such factors as "Western lifestyle" and its promotion of women's freedom, as well as "lack of financial security," overcrowded housing, alcoholism, and the reduction of their own moral authority by churches, apartheid, and exclusion from government health programs.

Donors enter this world, which they often don't understand, and offer incentives. Money rains down into poor countries, and government officials quickly learn where to place baskets to catch it. The appeal of endless cash is clear, but its workings on a day-to-day level are not. Indeed, they are among the most invisible aspects of the whole story. How exactly did Western money induce Uganda to jettison its life-saving program? The story detailed below provides a glimpse into how the pressure works. The publication of this story, according to a friend, may likely lead the U.S. government to black-ball me from future work, at least in AIDS, reproductive health, or any related field. If this happens, well, at least I have told the story.

The Day the Zambezi Ran Dry

In 2003, an American condom marketing company I will call X convinced Zambia to go along with a mass media campaign aimed at getting teenagers to use condoms. As is its fashion, X obtained a "request" for such a program, as if the Zambian government had suddenly on its own spotted a need for bold latex promotion. However, the TV and radio ads aimed at getting kids to use condoms provoked an outcry from religious leaders, parents, teachers, and society in general—and they would have anywhere. Not even the United States would have allowed such stuff on its airwaves. So X had to halt its campaign a few months after it was rolled out.

Urgent meetings took place between X and its Zambian partners.

It quickly became apparent the "partners" did not really represent the vox populi—the values, beliefs, and sentiments of the majority of Zambians. Rather, a group called SAGE (Stakeholders Advisory Group, Expanded) arose and eventually there was a compromise. The condom campaign could continue but only if there was a parallel and equal campaign promoting abstinence. When I arrived in Zambia in 2003, I found myself invited to a meeting of SAGE "stakeholders." Almost everybody at the meeting was connected to a USAID-funded project. There were also *mzungus* (whites). They included a European I'll call Marjorie from UNAIDS and a Canadian I'll call Tess from DFID (the Department for International Development, the UK's rough analogue to USAID). I saw one man from the Ugandan Central Board of Health. There was also an African program officer from the local NGO Family Health Trust, Mrs B. Other than the last, there was no voice representative of Zambian society, certainly none from any of the groups that would have objected to a condom ad on TV.

The new radio and TV spots had allegedly undergone a rigorous and fully participatory development process. At the meeting we would make the final decisions, approving ads or seeking revisions. It seemed that everyone at the meeting was a believer in condoms and a critic of abstinence. Two white women in particular raised multiple objections to abstinence elements, even in the abstinence ads—despite the fact that the campaign was now supposed to include them. One of the best ads was aimed at rural schoolgirls and contained the lines: "Are you crazy? You know you shouldn't be doing it. You should be abstaining." Marjorie objected because, she said, these sentences "stigmatized" those who couldn't abstain and were completely unrealistic. And so they vanished.

I wondered if Marjorie thought all criticism created stigma. I also wondered how much money had gone into (1) the original development of this ad, (2) the systematic focus groups conducted in three or four parts of the country, and (3) the eight-hour meeting the previous day with the Youth Advisory Group (YAG) made up of about fifty young people from various parts of Zambia. The message had passed all these hurdles, yet in the end, one Westerner disliked something, and out it went. Actually, even the condom-supporting Zambian employees of the project tried to explain that in Zambia, you couldn't just expect people to accept condoms. Most Zambian citizens would expect the abstinence message to come first, they argued, or at least to be mentioned before condoms. But the foreigners didn't listen and the lines that had upset Marjorie disappeared.

The UNAIDS woman was quite upset over one tag line: "Be strong, abstain from sex." She simply didn't like the message of abstaining. If we had to mention abstinence in every condom spot, she asked, why couldn't we mention condoms in every abstinence spot? Tess replied, "Politics." I heard this word several times in this meeting and the group understood that *politics alone* accounted for the abstinence message they were dealing with. Indeed, an observer from Mars would have heard a great deal of one viewpoint, and assuming this was a meeting of representative stakeholders, would have concluded that no Zambian wanted to delay sexual debut.

The group also discussed whether one could say that abstaining did more than "reduce" the risk of HIV infection. The previous day I had suggested expanding the message to "eliminate." Now I heard the counterargument: Because you could get HIV from a blood transfusion, abstaining reduced but did not eliminate the risk of infection. I almost laughed. Most Africans never even see a doctor, let alone have blood transfusions. But I was overruled, or thought I was. Surprisingly, Marjorie of UNAIDS sided with me, because "pregnancy" occurred in the same line. And UNAIDS argued that abstaining more than reduced the risk of pregnancy; it eliminated it. Because this suggestion came from someone with impeccable condom credentials, Tess agreed to change the wording from "reduce risk" of infection and pregnancy to "avoid risk."

In addition to the ease with which one or two whites can significantly alter a spot that's gone through a long, expensive participatory process, there was yet another problem. An American I'll call Bev introduced a TV ad in a way that preempted any critical feedback. It showed a broad river drying up, as well as a canoe and people hunting birds. The young YAG members had expressed concerns. What was the canoe supposed to mean? The river? Why birds? Were we supposed to believe that the Zambezi River dried up so that a person could walk across it? The Zambezi goes dry about as often as the Amazon. Now, before any stakeholder could comment, Bev stated emphatically that this TV spot was the most popular one in the focus groups. No one had found fault with any element of it, she protested defensively. Yet even with this discussion-killing introduction, people still wondered what this spot meant. It was clear that several hadn't a clue. The Zambian "facilitator" commented that few people hunt birds in Zambia; they hunt animals.

No reaction. He said it again: "We hunt animals." No reaction. I tried to help the group past this awkward moment, asking: "Do Zambians more often hunt for animals or birds?" Three Zambian men said in unison: "Animals." "In fact, antelope. Impala." Marjorie dismissed the comment. The *mzungus* had me squirming in my seat. So I suggested that this spot resembled another one built around basketball. A couple of YAG members had mentioned that Zambians knew soccer much better than basketball, so the spot had changed the sport mentioned. I suggested that the birds-versus-animals issue was similar. The American presenter Bev seemed upset and said, "Now we'll have to go through focus groups again." She had presented the findings from the focus groups like this: "Lusaka liked this spot. Livingstone didn't like that spot. Livingstone said use this line, while Lusaka said they are lukewarm on it." In other words, we heard that every focus group had a single viewpoint, as if it were a person.

After the meeting, I spoke to Mrs. B. Her group, Family Health Trust, is a true Zambian NGO, rather than one of those that sprout up as soon as AIDS funds become available. The trust began in 1987 and had established anti-AIDS Clubs in the primary schools, and a few secondary schools as well. The target group was young people from seven to seventeen, especially youth before debut. In other words, she was active on the ground, as I had been. She told me that she also was concerned that "people" (she was too polite to say *mzungus*) were watering down abstinence messages despite the elaborate and democratic Zambian design process. I asked what her AIDS prevention message was. Mrs. B. looked at me nervously and admitted that it was abstinence. When I didn't roll my eyes or make a sarcastic remark, she seemed to relax and began to speak more freely. The idea, she said, is to keep youth abstaining until marriage, although they didn't usually use "delay," as in Uganda; they used the controversial A-word. She said they didn't normally mention condoms, but when condom questions arise, they do discuss them. Finally, Mrs. B. said she thought today's meeting had been very biased, with no alternative viewpoints expressed. She knew that condoms were not all that protective, certainly not the "nearly 100 percent" that the USAID-funded organizations had been promoting.

I also met briefly with Marjorie and Tess before leaving the meeting. I asked why they thought prevalence had fallen among youth since the mid-1990s. Marjorie didn't hesitate: "It's the FBOs. For all their stigmatizing ways, they must be credited with pushing more abstinence." *Huh?* I thought. But then, a few minutes later, Marjorie was again saying that FBOs were valuable only to the extent that they promoted condoms. She had a "true story" to tell: The Catholic Youth Alive program pokes holes in condoms, then goes to schools to demonstrate their weaknesses. She said this makes her blood boil. Tess's mouth fell open in astonishment. Incidentally, Tess mentioned that the average age of first sex is about age eleven. I corrected her, and Marjorie backed me up: it is 16.6 for girls and about 17.5 for boys. The Canadian woman was amazed.

This was an evidence-informed approach in action.

The Upstairs, Downstairs of Foreign Aid

Remarkably, this meeting actually did entail some African feedback. Westerners often ignored it, but at least they heard it. Most of the time African feedback is simply absent. This problem afflicts not only HIV campaigns, but foreign aid in general. As surprising as it may sound, Westerners don't take the response on the ground seriously. A 2000 World Bank study concluded: "Despite the billions of dollars spent on development assistance each year, there is still very little known about the actual impact of [a] project on the poor." We address Third World problems too much with the donors at home in mind. They pay the bills. Imagine an *Upstairs, Downstairs*, where the aristocrats want to improve the lot of the servants. To carry out this task they hire go-betweens, who answer to the aristocrats. The latter rarely go downstairs themselves, and when they do, the go-betweens coordinate what they see and with whom they talk. If the aristocrats feel good about the efforts, they'll keep funding the go-betweens, regardless of actual conditions downstairs. That's pretty much the world of foreign aid.

Foreign aid has scored a few important victories, however—notably in health. For instance, foreign aid has ended smallpox and nearly eradicated polio and the loathsome guinea worm. It slashed childhood deaths from diarrhea in Egypt and trachoma in Morocco, and almost vanquished measles in southern Africa and river blindness in West Africa. These are plainly great achievements. Unfortunately, these instances stand out like stars against the blackness of failed attempts. I have spent an enormous part of my professional career on the ground, in places like Suriname and Swaziland, with people like the rain forest Matawai and the Swazi. I have seen foreign aid in operation and I have derived a development philosophy—if it can be called that—from long firsthand experience. I did not simply dream it up, devise it from books, or select it from a drop-down menu. I have learned this philosophy from nearly forty years of work in and out of less-developed countries.

In essence, it is this: *People don't want outsiders to come in and solve the problems.* They want the tools to solve them themselves. And those nations that have emerged from poverty over the past fifty years—such as Singapore, Taiwan, and increasingly China—have in fact done it alone. Consider Jamaica. In 1996 its government asked USAID if, instead of 80 percent or more of AIDS funds going to American "technical assistance" (read: U.S. personnel and technology), couldn't all the funds go directly to Jamaica? After all, they argued, Jamaica has good AIDS prevention people who knew their own culture better than outsiders. The U.S. could monitor every dollar spent on AIDS prevention, in a special account. To its credit, USAID agreed, and I had the great good luck to be one of three evaluators sent to Jamaica in 2000 to see what the nation had accomplished. We found that Jamaica had developed a program with many similarities to Uganda's original approach, and that infection rates seemed to have stabilized and were probably declining.

There are many reasons why outsider intervention tends not to work, but here are four:

1. *Ignorance.* Outsiders too often don't understand the problem. That's partly because "the problem" is often a million little interrelated problems.
2. *Overconfidence.* Outsiders too often think they do understand the problem. That's partly because they have more schooling than most Africans and have read more books and reports by authors who claim to get it. It's also because the most confident and persuasive outsiders tend to get the funding.
3. *Top-down approach.* Outsiders tend to arrive with big programs for overhaul, which also appeal to funders. Yet newly rich societies like Taiwan have grown organically, by making endless improvements throughout, such as forging commercial links and streamlining the flow of business. Outsiders replicate the mistake of communists. They think economies and

societies are systems manageable from above. In fact, they are vast, intricate, highly sensitive webs, and ultimately they have to develop by themselves. Outsiders can help, and certainly have, but they can hardly create these networks themselves.

4. *Perverse incentives.* Aid program workers are accountable to the upstairs donors at home, not to the people they are supposed to help. So they tend to measure success in dollars spent, not results. They also tend to focus on efforts easily communicated at home, such as condom distribution. If the Zambezi goes dry, for example, donors may remember it, even if Africans scoff.

On a more formal level, and other things being equal, I tend to favor solutions that are:

- Low-cost and based on self-help rather than reliant on government or bureaucratic services
- Self-sustainable rather than dependent
- Low-tech rather than high-tech
- Indigenous rather than Western
- Reflective of human beings in their higher roles, such as being responsible and ethical

Furthermore, these solutions:

- Show people as proactive rather than reactive victims of circumstance, and demonstrate the capacity for people to change their own behavior
- Expose the fallibility of widely admired and seldom questioned experts
- Show victories of common sense over professionalism and experts, of David over Goliath, of the Third World peasant over the Western technocrat

I see quite a bit of my own philosophy in the economist William Easterly's *The White Man's Burden* (2006). Easterly has challenged the ideas and practices of "utopian social engineering" by international development experts called Planners, for whom poverty is an engineering problem with technical solutions only they can concoct. He contrasts it with a type of expert we encounter far less often: Searchers, who go to Africa with humility, open minds, and an ability to learn what works in different cultural settings. Planners may become entrenched because donors have trouble identifying real success. "Goals are observable to the rich-country public while results are not," he notes, and hence donors tend to reward intent, not accomplishment.[7] In response, recipient organizations focus more on image than solution. For instance, a World Bank study found that money spent on Third World textbooks yields a payoff fourteen times greater than that on schoolhouses. Yet buildings are more visible than books, so they get the money. Agencies can take before-and-after photos—vacant land + funds = school—and donors can read glossy brochures that show happy children trooping in for class and teachers with pointers at blackboards. In this way we waste money and kids go uneducated. Substitute condoms for schoolhouses and fidelity for textbooks, and you have African AIDS.

To some extent, AIDS programs are responding to the same dynamics as most other foreign aid efforts, especially when they make common cause in goals like gender equality. They have adapted to the donor environment. It is hard to change course. We have underwritten risk reduction with billions of dollars, provided programs and bureaucracies with strong connections to family-planning organizations, and placed professional reputations, egos, and careers on the line. Contractors and grantees still benefit financially from the multibillion-dollar global AIDS industry and see no reason to endorse behavior change programs that can succeed without their medical products and services.

Yet change is possible.

PART IV

SHIFTING THE RIVERBED

A liberal is someone who opposes interference in the affairs of others: who is tolerant of dissenting attitudes and unconventional behavior. . . . Most genuine liberals remain disposed to leave other people alone.

TONY JUDT
Ill Fares the Land

I began to feel that I was living in a strange world, one in which the plainest of truths before one's nose could neither be said out loud nor in any way acknowledged. It therefore seemed to partake of the atmosphere of Kafka.

THEODORE DALRYMPLE
Romancing the Opiates

It is sometimes important for science to know how to forget the things she is surest of.

JEAN ROSTAND
Reflections of a Biologist

CHAPTER 8

Jihad

By 2001 I had declared war against this massive superstructure of thought and practice, and I had taken the first step by signing a book contract. But I remained more or less a lone individual, and I had a few entanglements. The previous year I had served on the board of directors of the World Population Society, along with Henry Cole, my old boss from Social Marketing for Change (SOMARC), a program under The Futures Group. Henry and a sweet octogenarian named Page Wilson—who had been press agent to JFK's dad Joe when he was U.S. ambassador to the UK—were quite interested in my message about behavior change and the role of faith-based organizations (FBOs) in AIDS prevention. Before long, Henry asked if I would come back to work at Futures, to help change the thinking there.

I was reluctant, mainly because I had developed a terrific professional life as an independent consultant. I was taking assignments on every continent but Antarctica, and I continued to publish scholarly articles as well as books. But finally I relented, agreeing to work half-time at Futures. I hoped to interest its AIDS experts in my findings and help them think differently—futuristically—about how behavior change could bring Futures more grants and contracts. For the other 50 percent of my time, I would keep consulting hither and yon. Several months passed at The Futures Group. I quickly realized that the AIDS experts there were inhospitable to my ideas and findings. This was awkward. I really liked Henry and I felt I owed him quite a bit for all the good things he'd done for me over the years. He really wanted my ideas to catch on at Futures, but they just weren't. How was I going to get out of this situation?

A few weeks after signing my book contract, my wife Suzie and I were in Maine, and she said, "Now that we've inherited your family property, isn't there some way we can spend more time up here?"

"Well, Sooze," I said. "I'm a consultant and that means I have to be in D.C., where all the international action originates. The belly of the beast and all that . . ."

"But what if you could get a job at, say, Harvard?" she asked. "Wouldn't that be worth moving up here for?" Especially, she added, if I was going to expose a billion-dollar industry. She thought Ted Green, Harvard U., would carry more weight than Ted Green, Independent Consultant. But how could I get to Harvard at age fifty-six, after being a nonacademic applied anthropologist for some twenty-five years? Many well-known career scholars never even got close to its fabled ivy.

A few days later, I was online reading a listserv about African health issues. I didn't usually follow it, and never before (or since) had I seen it advertise a postdoc program of any sort. But now I saw a listing about a fellowship program for late middle-age paradigm bashers at the Harvard School of Public Health. (The language of the Takemi Post-Doc Fellowship actually reads more like: "For those scholars in mid-career who already have an independent research program with potential to impact international health policy.") Harvard was actually calling. But the due date for applications and proposals was Friday.

Hmm. It was Tuesday. I knew my proposal would not be popular, or even acceptable. But I thought, *What the hell?*

I fired off an e-mail to the Takemi folks proposing to write a book detailing the world's errors in AIDS prevention, especially in Africa. The standard formula of condoms-testing-drugs had failed, I declared, yet fidelity had succeeded. I stated frankly that this idea had "politically incorrect" branded on its forehead in steaming letters and had met strong resistance from experts. However, if Harvard thought it was worth a shot, I needed a deadline extension, partly because I had to round up letters of recommendation for the first time in decades. Consultants get assignments based on reputation and personal networks. The Takemi program wrote back to say that my idea sounded "interesting" and that I could take an extra week if I needed it. (I later found out that this response had come from a rather low-level administrator and that the head of the program seemed quite astonished when I showed up and told him the topic of my book.)

I then promptly left for a fascinating assignment in the Philippines, evaluating its national AIDS program with another well-known maverick in the field, Dr. Jim Chin of the University of California at Berkeley. Jim is a short Chinese American, in his late sixties back then, and he talks just like Woody Allen. He had even grown up in the same neighborhood and attended the same school as Allen. We got along great. One day in Manila, I received an e-mail telling me that Harvard had accepted my postdoc proposal. I ate dinner with Jim that night and asked if he thought I should take it. "Hell, yes!" he said, you can stir things up.

Back in Academia

You need a lot more than a Harvard position to unmask a multibillion-dollar industry. First, you require a certain naïveté and hubris. To show how politically innocent I was, I'll recount this near humiliating event: I was on stage at Johns Hopkins University debating AIDS prevention with the comprehensive sex education guru Doug Kirby. A student directed a rather hostile question at me from the floor: "What about the special needs of LGBTQ?" "Er . . . excuse me," I stammered. Mercifully, Doug whispered to me: "She means lesbian, gay, bisexual, transgendered, and 'questioning' or queer."

("Intersexual" has since been added, at least in South Africa.) Kirby saved me from mortification. Who did I think I was, being in a debate on a college campus and not knowing the lingo?

At Harvard I soon discovered the powerful force of the pressure against a diversity of ideas. Universities encourage innovation in myriad important ways, but the pressures to conform to broader modes of thinking are almost overpowering. Earlier in my career I had challenged leading anthropologists of the past seventy-five years in my book *Indigenous Theories of Contagious Disease* (1999), and I never worried that peers would reject me or that I would lose my job. I had ties to too many organizations, none run by anthropologists. Mine was the attitude of someone working independently and alone, outside the academy, for many years. Being at Harvard made me realize just how good I'd had it as a free-ranging consultant and scholar, pre-2001. Just the right environment to take on the Whole Damned System, with few inhibitions! If my writing challenges many politically correct ideas, it is to some extent because I was in the field practicing anthropology and had almost no academic connections between 1979 and 2001.

I spent 2001 and 2002 working on my book and speaking out as much as possible. I teamed up with the Ugandan infectious disease specialist Vinand Nantulya, first at Harvard and later at the Global Fund. Vinand had been a Takemi Fellow the previous year. Harvard liked him so much that he was staying on, doing research on road safety in the Third World. The head of the Takemi program thought highly of Vinand and so I ran my ideas past him. It turned out that we saw the problem in Uganda in exactly the same way. It also turned out that President Museveni had phoned his old friend Vinand back in 1986, soon after receiving the urgent alert from Fidel Castro. Museveni had asked Vinand to return to Uganda and advise him on handling this deadly new plague. Vinand had been present at the outset. Vinand and I would often speak together, including on Voice of America TV, broadcast in several African countries. USAID

also funded us to conduct research on the relative merits of the elements of the ABC approach (abstain, be faithful, or use a condom)
in six countries.

After my Takemi year (2001–02), I joined the Center for Population and Development Studies at Harvard. Its director, Michael Reich,
got me an initial three-year appointment to allow me more time to
finish the book. He also thought that I, perhaps along with Vinand,
could take leadership roles at establishing a broad, universitywide
AIDS prevention initiative. He asked me to help sort out problems
with a fifty-million-dollar AIDS prevention effort in Nigeria, funded
by the Bill and Melinda Gates Foundation. Although "prevention"
was right there in the project title, apparently no one had undertaken
any form of prevention to date (and it was not Michael's fault because
he had just joined the effort). So what would we tell the foundation
when the project finished? We'd just been *thinking* about prevention? Or: prevention wasn't possible, so we'd spent the money as we
pleased? The endeavor had just a year or two left when Michael asked
me to spend 10 percent of my time advising it. I was happy to try.

The director of this research was an evolutionary virologist who
actually did think AIDS was unpreventable. Yet she seemed happy to
engage groups of Nigerian professors in scholarly issues. I described
the matter quite bluntly to Michael, and he chuckled and suggested
that I might try to find a more . . . um, *diplomatic* way to give advice.
He said it would be better if I came up with specific suggestions.

A while later, Michael told me that a group of professors from
Ibadan University, colleagues on this project, was coming to Harvard. We thought their visit might be a good occasion to present
my ideas about African AIDS prevention, Uganda-style. The day
finally arrived, and Vinand and I each gave a slide presentation. I
said, "Gentlemen, we still have a year and a half left. Why don't we
promote behavior change through religious organizations, because
Uganda did it so successfully, and these groups are eager to collaborate." There was a momentary stillness, as if I'd told them Nigeria

had just become the fifty-first American state. Then one professor after another remarked that the idea actually sounded great, and come to think of it, why no one had mentioned this to them before? Nigerians are "very religious people," they pointed out, and this strategy would probably be highly effective at bringing messages of behavior change to the masses. In my experience Africans *always* think involving Christian and Muslim leaders is a good idea.

Over the remaining months of the project, the professors insisted that we carry out a national KAP ("knowledge, attitudes, and practices") survey that would give us a sense of Nigerian sexual behavior, awareness of HIV, and knowledge of condoms. I told them this survey was unnecessary because there had already been many such studies in Nigeria. For instance, Dr. Jack Caldwell and his team of Australian and international researchers had studied sexual networks in Nigeria and left a body of literature unparalleled on the continent. But no, they wanted to do their *own* study. I argued that by the time we carried out a study, the project would be over and all we'd have to show for the fifty-million-dollar foundation grant would be another KAP study.

And that, dear reader, is pretty much what happened.

To Washington

Meanwhile, a brilliant anthropologist named Daniel Halperin had become a supporter. Unlike me, Daniel had had formal training in public health, including epidemiology, at UC Berkeley. He wanted to do the kind of work I was doing, and we were allies on two crucial issues: ABC and male circumcision. There were a few other backers of male circumcision in the 1990s, but essentially none for fidelity or partner reduction. I helped Daniel get a few crucial consulting assignments with organizations funded by USAID. Then a dream job opened up at USAID headquarters: Global Adviser on AIDS and Behavior Change. Daniel applied for it, and I wrote a very strong letter of support, citing his recent experience evaluating AIDS programs as a consultant. Daniel landed the job and then went about trying to convert the USAID Office of HIV/AIDS and the Office of Family Planning to our way of understanding African AIDS.

We needed a kickoff event. So he arranged for me to come down to USAID headquarters and give a presentation billed as "What Happened in Uganda?" I was a little anxious about this whole affair, in part because I knew the audience would greet my ideas with hostility and counterattack. I knew someone would make me admit during Q&A that my field experience in Uganda was measured in weeks and months, not years; that person might then say that he or she had spent ten or twenty years there and I had the story all wrong. I had the perfect idea: my new friend Vinand would come down to Washington, D.C., with me. Some folks at USAID were already learning about my views and getting nervous. They insisted that if "this Green" would be talking, AIDS and condom specialist John Stover (from The Futures Group, no less!) also had to attend to argue that everyone had been right all along.

We gave our speeches, as did John. As expected, there was hostility in the audience, but it would have been bad form to attack an African about events in his own country, so it was muted. Later, a smattering of people in the audience, including some from Johns Hopkins, actually came up to tell me (well, *whisper*) that this approach to AIDS prevention was the best they'd ever heard. Somehow the whole affair was videotaped and the Voice of America played the presentations in Kenya, Uganda, and elsewhere.

Around this time a small group of us—Daniel and me, Vinand, Rand Stoneburner and Daniel Low-Beer, and a bit later Norman Hearst (the epidemiologist at the University of California) and science journalist Helen Epstein—began exchanging e-mails about what worked and didn't work in AIDS prevention. We discussed intriguing questions that most AIDS researchers seemed to be ignoring, such as why AIDS had skyrocketed in Africa despite the fact that Africans had fewer sex partners in a lifetime and less premarital sex than people in the West. It was a smart, exciting private forum, and at times we had ten or more illuminating exchanges in a single day. Occasionally, freethinker Jim Chin joined us, but he agreed with us mainly about the grossly inflated figures for HIV prevalence that everyone was using, rather than about the fidelity factor or male circumcision.

This group also discussed the landmark 2003 UNAIDS study on condom effectiveness by Hearst and his graduate student Sanny Chen. Hearst had recently done a controlled community trial in Uganda to measure the impact of super-intense condom promotion and provision. He tried to get a last-minute abstract into the global AIDS conference in Barcelona in 2004, but he was a few days too late. He is now grateful for that, because his same findings would show later that intense condom promotion actually leads to riskier behavior and probably higher HIV infection rates. If he had presented those findings, UNAIDS never would have hired him to do his key study of condom effectiveness. They *did* hire him, however: he was to review all high-quality studies and reach conclusions that would make UNAIDS and the rest of the industry happy.

What they didn't know is that Norman is an honest man and a careful scientist. He and Chen presented their results to UNAIDS, and they were not what that agency was expecting. The authors had "found no evidence that condoms alone have played a major role in HIV prevalence decline, anywhere in Africa." So UNAIDS did what the World Bank did to my 1998 report: they pretended it had never happened. But Norman detailed the findings in an article and submitted it to the *Journal of Acquired Immune Deficiency Syndrome (JAIDS)*. It was quickly rejected. Meanwhile, he had sent drafts of the paper to me, Daniel, Jim Shelton (a top adviser in the Office of Family Planning with USAID), and others, hoping to find the most nonthreatening language possible yet still remain faithful to the truth. After twice the normal number and length of peer reviewers, the basic findings appeared in *Studies in Family Planning* (not an AIDS journal, but close).[1]

Of course, after this publication of the basic findings, people began contacting UNAIDS to see the full study results. UNAIDS crafted a summary that managed to ignore the most important find- ings. This is the kind of corruption of science that would have had me threatening lawsuits and calling in the commandos. But Norman is a patient, low-keyed scientist who will doubtless live longer than I will. He observed that although the UN did ignore 90 percent of the findings, they nevertheless mentioned 10 percent, and "10 percent is better than no percent, right?"

The USAID ABC Study

Using his position at USAID, Daniel Halperin managed to find funds for a study to examine the relative contributions of ABC fac- tors to HIV prevalence decline. Was it really little A, big B, and little C, as some of us freethinkers suspected? We could now find out. The most senior USAID person involved in our study was Jim Shelton, who advised in the Office of Family Planning, not HIV/AIDS. Still, he was a condom expert and we needed such a high-level backer. Someone from MACRO International, the company that conducts the Demographic and Health Survey (DHS) studies related to contra- ception and AIDS, was to be the principal investigator of Phase I of the ABC Study. I myself would be the principal investigator of Phase II, which would involve fieldwork in six countries. We would select three "successful" countries in AIDS prevention and three unsuc- cessful ones. A Memo of Understanding was written and signed, affirming that we could follow the evidence wherever it led us.

Because Vinand and I had said at our USAID presentation that we thought fidelity explained Uganda's success better than condoms, we were widely thought of as biased. Because so many people supported condoms, the idea of a pro-condom bias apparently never occurred to anyone. Bias, like ideology, was something other people had. From the pre-AIDS era of family planning, critics of condoms were branded as Catholic or Evangelical conservatives. Therefore, those of us who raised questions about the efficacy of condoms in AIDS prevention were likewise dismissed as being motivated by religion or politics. In any case, USAID went to great lengths to counter my alleged bias. First, to administer the contract, USAID selected PSI, an organization that began by selling porn sex videos and dildos and later morphed into the biggest condom social marketer on earth. The first study to look objectively at the relative contribution of condoms would take place under the authority of the company with the most at stake in the results. Second, we had originally agreed that all six countries would be in Africa, but now we learned that one of the three successes would be Thailand. Thailand was becoming famous as a great triumph of condoms, so in case the devices looked bad in Africa, Thailand could cushion the damage. USAID biased the study in other egregious ways, and I detailed them in a confidential memo, in case this ever became a legal matter.

Nevertheless, I was being offered an opportunity to stay on at Harvard if I could get grant money, and here was grant money. Also, my book was taking longer than I had expected, in part because the deeper I looked into AIDS World, the more mirages I found. But some excellent opportunities also arose during my Takemi year and the following years at the Harvard Center for Population and Development Studies (my affiliation there was from 2002 through May 2010). For example, the USAID mission in Kampala invited me over as part of a team to determine Uganda's needs going forward. As I described earlier, I found powerful evidence that USAID (with the help of the CDC and a host of other Western donor organizations) was doing almost *everything wrong* there. They were bulldozing Uganda's unique and highly effective program into rubble. I made some permanent enemies during that trip, especially because a British guy from the UN who had just joined USAID seemed to support my views, as did all Ugandans I consulted. But I was also getting some great, up-to-date evidence for the book.

In 2003, I went down to Washington, D.C., with Vinand and a

third Harvard scholar, Dr. Yaa Oppong, to present our preliminary findings. This time the audience was larger. It included not just the handful of USAID officers directly involved in the ABC Study, but important people who were highly alarmed, especially by some comments from Vinand. Soon after, USAID announced it was replacing me with a new principal investigator. *What about the memo of understanding? Did it have phrases in invisible ink? Did it say, "The investigators can follow the evidence wherever it leads,* but USAID can fire them if they do"?

The new principal investigator was no typical African AIDS expert; in fact, he had no expertise in Africa or anywhere outside the United States. It was Doug Kirby, widely reviled by some religious conservatives for opposing abstinence programs and championing "comprehensive sex education." In their eyes Kirby was not just a condom lover and an abstinence hater; he was a demon who reported directly to Satan. So I quit the study. Before USAID could respond, conservative supporters told me they were prepared to have the administration intervene. The White House would call the USAID administrator and have Kirby fired before he was hired, and I would be principal investigator again.

But they would only do it if I wanted to confront the situation head-on. I said I didn't. Let them take Kirby aboard and see what happens. It was well known that USAID had awarded the grant to me, through Harvard, and that the written understanding guaranteed a free investigation. Doug Kirby turned out to be intellectually honest. He assembled his own team and went to Uganda to get a clear picture of what happened there. Left to his own devices, he more or less validated what I had said all along: that partner reduction was the key to success in Uganda. In 2008, Kirby ultimately published his results in the journal *Sexually Transmitted Infections* and gave more credit to condoms than I would have, but otherwise we were not far apart.[2]

Sometime between 2004 and 2005, Kirby and I offered to write a joint report. Considering all the fireworks (for example, the highest-ranking health officer at USAID was basically fired for the perception that she mishandled the ABC Study), we thought our collaboration could help calm and heal the situation. Certainly both of us could contribute to useful AIDS prevention knowledge. After all, a study funded by taxpayers is supposed to yield a report those taxpayers can read. But fear and tensions were still running so high that USAID declined the offer of a two-author document, or any kind of document for that matter. I presented my detailed findings in *Rethinking AIDS Prevention*, and Kirby published his in the *Sexually Transmitted Infections* article. I am actually happy with the way things turned out, and I think the whole tale is illuminating: One researcher gets replaced by another for political reasons, and the other researcher then ignores the politics and comes up with essentially the same findings. They become colleagues and even friends as a result.

In December 2005, Kirby and I had the public debate at Johns Hopkins University I mentioned earlier. The auditorium was full of AIDS experts, including big shots from USAID, as well as the former director of its Office of Family Planning. Kicking off the affair, I tried to ease the tension with a little jest: "Well, you're all here to hear the contrasting views of Ted Green and Doug Kirby. Actually, I had Thanksgiving dinner at Kirby's house in California a few weeks ago, and we found out that we've come to agree on all the essential points. So I guess you can all go home (heh-heh)!" There was muted chuckling, but I am sure no one believed it was pretty much the truth. I presented my findings. I was eager to quote someone else in the audience, the science journalist Helen Epstein. She had recently made an excellent comment about the importance of reducing multiple partners. Now, I had made the same point far earlier, but I often found myself preferring to quote someone else, just to show I was not alone in my heresy.

Kirby then presented his findings. I remember thinking, *Doug and I are way ahead of this high-powered audience. I wonder if they can hear us back there.*

CHAPTER 9

Breakthrough

When I declared a jihad on the AIDS racket, I swore I'd do whatever it took to expose the truth. That meant reaching out to the Bush administration despite my political differences with it. In 2002, President Bush called his AIDS czar Joe O'Neill, an openly gay physician from Johns Hopkins, to the White House to discuss an example of "compassionate conservatism." The president wanted to save children by treating HIV-infected mothers with a single dose of neveripine.[1] O'Neill was delighted that Bush wanted to take action on AIDS, but he pointed out that a public-health approach would require placing drug treatment on a strong foundation of AIDS *prevention*. "Whoa," went the Bush advisers. "You're not gonna ask us to endorse condoms and syringes, are you?" No. O'Neill or someone told them there was a Harvard scientist named Green who had actually shown that abstaining and being faithful worked better than condoms, at least in Africa.

I was developing a national reputation around this time, and now, near the end of 2002, I was invited on an official trip to Uganda with Claude Allen, a conservative black lawyer who was then deputy secretary of the Department of Health and Human Services. After the trip I wrote a memo to Dr. Anne Peterson, the global health administrator at USAID, laying out our findings. I stressed the importance of fidelity and delay. A week later USAID reversed itself on fidelity and publicly stated that it was largely responsible for the Uganda turnaround. It also adopted the ABC program (abstain, be faithful, or use a condom) as the official U.S. strategy for the generalized epidemics of Africa, and this "Uganda ABC Approach" used much language taken directly from my writings or presentations. A cable went out signed by the secretary of state Colin Powell on December 31, 2002, affirming the new policy. I felt a shift in the AIDS universe.

The next month came a jolt. In January 2003, President Bush surprised the world in his State of the Union address by announcing his intention to battle AIDS in Africa. "We have a chance to achieve a more compassionate world for every citizen," he stated. "America believes deeply that everybody has worth, everybody matters, everybody was created by the Almighty, and we're going to act on that belief and we'll act on that passion." He also said that faith-based organizations would get some of the money. That same month he revealed the President's Emergency Plan for AIDS Relief (PEPFAR), a fifteen-billion-dollar program to fight the disease in Africa and the Caribbean. Of this sum, 55 percent went to treatment, 15 percent to palliative care of victims, 10 percent to aid for orphans, and 20 percent to prevention. Ultimately, it allocated a third of all prevention funds—or 7 percent of the total—to abstinence *and* fidelity. But it was a big total. Congress passed it in May, and PEPFAR had taken effect by June of 2004.

PEPFAR sparked jubilation at UNAIDS and elsewhere. In 1999 President Clinton had wrangled Congress into boosting global AIDS funding from $125 million up to $225 million. Bush had seemed oblivious to AIDS, but now he was increasing that amount by sixty-seven times. What had changed? Elizabeth Pisani credits the bill to the ultra-conservative senator Jesse Helms and his sudden shift from condemnation to concern about AIDS. Others speculated that prime movers were the senator Bill Frist and the Rev. Franklin Graham, and suggested that Bush had deployed the plan to counter the bloodshed in Iraq with mercy and healing. But I heard the impetus for prevention had come from Dr. O'Neill and my ABC advocacy.

PEPFAR spawned a typhoon. AIDS World and its many allies predicted mass death, especially in Africa. They misrepresented ABC as "abstinence-only" and spread the notion far and wide that it was "scientifically proven" not to work. Many critics claimed there was right-wing congressional support for "abstinence-and-faithfulness programs." In fact, no one supported fidelity. I tried to tell Republicans (as did Daniel Halperin at USAID) that they were starting on the wrong foot, fighting for abstinence over fidelity. They responded, in essence: "There is a *constituency* for abstinence. We haven't really thought about fidelity."

"The A-word, abstinence, has become a political lightning rod," I told the *New York Times* (which called me "a hot property among conservatives in Washington these days"—how ironic!). "As soon as my colleagues hear it, they say, 'This is the Bush administration moralizing.' I wish we didn't even have that word in our vocabulary." I also wrote an op-ed for the *Times* in which I highlighted fidelity and pointed out that neither side had allied itself with the best strategy. "We need to develop a balanced approach," I wrote, "by recognizing that Africa and the West have different types of epidemics and going beyond the fruitless battle between the abstinence and condom camps."[2]

After that piece appeared, a number of people contacted me. One of the more interesting was Gabriel Rotello, who had written the provocative book *Sexual Ecology* in 1997.[3] Rotello is an openly gay science journalist, and his book hammered home the same message as my *Rethinking AIDS Prevention:* people need to behave responsibly and not have multiple concurrent sexual partners if they want to avoid AIDS. He observed that gay men—at least "fast-lane" urban gays— had developed self-damaging values and behavior patterns as well as mental screens against the self-scrutiny that might lead to safer behavior. Rotello asked if I had heard of his book. I told him I had a whole section on him appearing in my own book and that I really respected his courage. He and I have since taken occasional comfort in exchanging commiserative e-mails. We have both experienced similar stigma as traitors, but I'm pretty sure he was treated even worse than I was.

The President's Council

Overall, despite the political apathy toward fidelity, its inclusion in PEPFAR was revolutionary. Up until this time no interventions funded by major donors anywhere had aimed at limiting concurrent sex partners or delaying sexual "careers." In early 2003 I was invited to Washington, D.C., to brief the USAID administrator, White House officials, members of Congress, and senators and their staff. I made two formal presentations to Congress. A draft of my book circulated before publication, and I was asked to join the Presidential Advisory Council on HIV and AIDS (PACHA). I was also invited to be on OARAC (the Office of AIDS Research Advisory Council) under the National Institutes of Health (NIH). My papers and presentations were quoted widely. I coauthored an op-ed for the *Washington Post* and the *New York Times*. The *Chicago Tribune* and other media interviewed me, and PEPFAR the bill grew into PEPFAR the organization.

PACHA always met in Washington, D.C., usually at the headquarters of the Department of Health and Human Services. I now had high-level access and I could influence policy directly. *This is applied anthropology at its best*, I thought. I had a good experience on this committee. Its members were usually willing to look at the evidence objectively and find common ground. My major contribution was to get fellow council members to look at fundamental behavior change, at eliminating risk rather than reducing it. I ended up serving on the council for somewhat longer than the maximum allowable period. I formed some useful strategic alliances, notably with the African-American contingent, with Hank McKinnell (then the CEO of Pfizer), and other key individuals.

McKinnell asked me to talk with him, so we had dinner one night. He had said in his invitation: "In God we trust. All others bring evidence." I told him about Uganda during that dinner and he told me understanding the world's first success story was sufficiently important that he had Pfizer fund its own study, through Makerere University. Now, you'd think the biggest drug company on the planet would want to see AIDS prevention dependent on drugs and medical devices. If there was bias, it would be in that direction. But Hank McKinnell seemed a straight, honest guy, and the Pfizer study (released in August 2003) pretty much corroborated what I had told PACHA.[4] McKinnell became an ally.

McKinnell and I, along with one or two members, criticized PACHA for being far more reactive than proactive. At one fateful meeting during my third year on PACHA, McKinnell said, "Why don't we ask ourselves what it would take to bring the rate of new HIV infections in the world down to zero? In other words, putting aside financial and political considerations, and that includes political correctness, exactly what would we need to do?" I strongly seconded this idea and urged that we actually do this exercise. I pleaded for not carrying on business-as-usual, which meant liberals would bring in liberals to make formal presentations, and conservatives would bring in conservatives to make formal presentations. I argued that we had enough knowledge and experience among the thirty-odd souls sitting around the table. We were M.D.'s and Ph.D.'s, professors and government officials, minority AIDS activists, gays and straights, and here and there a recovering heroin addict. A good mix.

So that's just what we did. In December 2005 we produced a book called *Achieving an HIV-Free Generation*, available online at PACHA's Web site.[5] Among our recommendations were working with faith-based organization (FBOs), basing prevention on proven successes like Uganda, increasing male circumcision, providing more evidence-based preventive education, and collecting and reporting data better to replicate best practices. The only drugs recommended were those to prevent mother-to-child transmission. It was all very feet-on-the-ground. Every strategy was achievable. Remarkably, although cost was no object in this exercise, none of the recommendations was very expensive.

A Showcase of AIDS Africa

In December 2003, Tommy Thompson, then the U.S. Secretary of Health and Human Services, invited me to travel as part of an AIDS-related delegation to four African countries. The star-studded group included Thompson and myself as well as Ambassador Richard Holbrooke; Randall Tobias (the new head of PEPFAR, a position often called "global AIDS coordinator" or "AIDS ambassador"); the directors of the NIH, the CDC, WHO, and the Global Fund; the scientist Tony Fauci; Sen. Don Nickles (R-OK); Rep. Dave Weldon (R-FL); Hank McKinnell; and the CEOs of other major drug companies. I got invited because of my position on PACHA, and probably because of my role in persuading PEPFAR to adopt the ABC program.

My *Rethinking AIDS Prevention* was published just before this trip, in November 2003. It became a topic of conversation among the delegates. Richard Holbrooke rapid-read it on our chartered plane to Africa, and he got quite excited about the overlooked fidelity factor. He agreed with my critique of condoms, and persuaded Randy Tobias to read the book. It led to spirited discussions about what does and does not work in AIDS prevention. During a bus ride between Entebbe and Kampala, Tobias and I were midway in one such discussion when Dr. Anne Peterson of USAID joined in. Mark Dybul also participated, and in 2006, when he succeeded Randy as global AIDS coordinator, he proved a thoughtful and articulate defender of behavioral AIDS prevention. It was the perfect opportunity (no interruptions) and informal setting to discuss the most compelling evidence for Uganda's success against HIV.

Holbrooke said he was ready to endorse my book if I would fix one obvious shortcoming: I should make it clear that voluntary counseling and testing (VCT) was the other major solution besides fidelity. I told him that, as much as I would appreciate his endorsement, the evidence for VCT as a preventive measure just wasn't there. Maybe it would arise later, but we couldn't make that claim now. The next day we marched in the World AIDS Day parade in Livingstone, Zambia, and Holbrooke walked aside me, arguing that everyone on the trip was saying VCT was essential, so what's wrong with me? What did I have against testing? I told him: "Look, testing is essential for getting HIV-positive people into *treatment*, but not necessarily for prevention, as far as we can tell."

VCT was the next big thing at that moment. Organizations were broadening their emphasis from condoms to VCT, while still striving to keep the condom commerce robust. As Holbrooke was hearing it, the heads of the major AIDS and science organizations were maintaining that people would not change sexual behavior unless they knew their HIV status. If you realized you were positive, the thinking went, you wouldn't infect others. Many believed that people would change behavior no matter which way they tested. However, traditional HIV testing can't identify people in the super-contagious stage right after infection, before antibodies are visible. Two studies had already shown that VCT led to no behavior change in rural Uganda.[6] Several more in Africa showed that VCT did not affect the infection rate.[7] In fact, Ron Gray of Johns Hopkins had found that VCT *did* change behavior—for the worse. Gray, J. K. Motovu, and colleagues were among the first to burst the VCT bubble. They observed there was some evidence that VCT could improve condom use among those who tested positive. But they also found that it seemed to breed riskier behavior. When people repeatedly test negative, they tend to think that they're either hard to infect or very skilled at choosing partners. Sexual behavior becomes "disinhibited."[8] These were important findings, but like so many other investigators, he had trouble getting them published.

A 2010 study I conducted using Demographic and Health Survey data from Swaziland, Tanzania, and Zambia with Alison Ruark, Hearst, and Esther Hudes provides even more evidence. We found that married people who test HIV-positive are more likely to use condoms consistently, but unmarried males who test HIV-positive are not. These results undermine the many claims that African men will not protect their wives. We also found that testing HIV-negative did not increase condom use in most cases, and in Swaziland unmarried HIV-negative women reported significantly less consistent condom usage than unmarried women who had never been tested.[9] Despite this evidence, I doubt the AIDS industry will want to surrender counseling and testing. They serve critical purposes, without question, but one factor makes them especially appealing: the price tag. A comparative study of the different costs per case of HIV prevented found that the combination of counseling and testing was the most expensive nondrug method, at around four hundred to five hundred dollars per infection averted.[10] It's expensive because it involves one-on-one counseling, and the counseling is rarely about anything other than condom use.

Holbrooke didn't change his mind back then, and I could see why. In brief addresses later, Richard Feachem of the Global Fund and Tony Fauci had both claimed: "We *know* people will not change their behavior until they know their HIV status," hence everyone had to get tested ASAP. They spoke as if we actually had evidence to back up the position—rather as administration officials had about weapons of mass destruction in Iraq. By the way, Holbrooke remained very friendly to me, and he's an extremely bright and engaging guy. He used to work under my father, as deputy assistant secretary of state for East Asia and Pacific. He told a few stories about my mother who, bless her heart, liked to run everyone's lives for them, fixing my lifelong antipathy toward authority.

Given our sway, the "coalition of the billing" had a tight timeline ready for us, perhaps especially in Uganda. Our schedule and presentations brimmed over with condoms, drugs, testing, and various studies of vaccines and vaginal gels. No mention of behavior. No mention of ABC, even though it was now U.S. government policy. If a few others and I hadn't spoken out, the delegation would have left Uganda hearing nothing about the program that had made the nation so extraordinary. By 2003, Ugandans knew what donors favored: medical devices, drugs, and big clinical or prospective studies. Certainly these were the interests of the Americans working for USAID and the CDC. In fact, because the Uganda ABC model was so intensely unpopular with most U.S. personnel working in AIDS, local Americans were doing what they could to discredit it.

After my complaints to the U.S. ambassador to Uganda, Jimmy Kolker, and the minister of health, some meetings on abstinence were hastily arranged. But fidelity was harder. How do you inspect fidelity programs if there aren't any? One day, half our delegation went to a primary school to see an abstinence program. When I asked the headmaster what he was going to tell these super-delegates, I found he had not thought to mention that his abstinence program descended directly from one that UNICEF and others had developed in the 1980s. He agreed with my suggestion to add this information. I didn't want the group to think that the program before their eyes had sprung from the mind of George W. Bush.

Randy Tobias was in this group, sitting in the front row before fifty or so charming boys and girls, perhaps ages ten to fourteen, in yellow T-shirts that proclaimed their decision to abstain. Almost as soon as I met Tobias, I could see he was a quiet, sensitive, diplomatic, and caring guy, and these qualities shone here. In the first part of the program, set up in advance without our knowledge, he sat on a tiny stool on a school auditorium stage, fielding questions from the children. Tobias had been the CEO of the large pharmaceutical company Eli Lilly, but I don't know if he had any experience handling public interrogation from third-graders. Yet he seemed completely relaxed and genuinely interested in the children's questions. He gave sincere answers in a fatherly sort of way that did not speak down to the kids. I think everyone who witnessed this exercise in Lilliputian diplomacy was greatly impressed.

The children sang beautiful songs and we interviewed several of them. I have always believed that Africans are natural public speakers, even the kids. (I have yet to meet an African with a public-speaking phobia, which so many of my colleagues suffer from.) Their stories could not have been more moving if the Hollywood experts had scripted them. A few of the women with me in the audience actually wept softly at times. I looked at Tobias a few times and I could tell that he was deeply affected. I heard later that Tobias told people back in the State Department, and at USAID, that he really came to understand abstinence during this trip to Uganda. But of course he never experienced such an "aha" moment with fidelity. There was no program to visit to understand fidelity. There were no billboards for the delegates to see, and no radio or TV programs. Few if any Ugandans raised the subject voluntarily. Local officials and NGO heads knew what Western donors wanted, and it wasn't zero grazing.

The most unforgettable event for us all was probably the field trip to remote rural villages in the Tororo district. There we visited families where HIV-positive patients have been receiving antiretroviral drugs for several months, delivered by health workers on motorcycles. Some of the infected had, in their own words, come back from the threshold of death. They were full of enthusiasm for life and grateful to America for supplying the drugs, through a CDC-supported pilot program. Some delegates used this occasion to stress that counseling and testing were essential to AIDS prevention.

On our last evening in Africa I was invited to make a fifteen-minute speech to the whole delegation. I urged that in our excitement over finally bringing life-saving antiretrovirals to Africa's poor, we not neglect AIDS prevention. I mentioned that ARVs could lead to riskier sexual behavior, as they had among gay men in the United States. I stressed that, with the recent adoption of the ABC program, we could finally prevent AIDS more effectively, and I told them about Ugandans' extraordinary past success with fidelity. But they only had my word for it.

The Consensus Statement

The decision makers had seen only one kind of evidence on the ground in Uganda, and the facts had been hard enough to find that my book was a revelation to many of them. Yet 2004 became a watershed year in academic and medical journals; studies about Uganda and fidelity finally had made it past peer review. That year leading scientific journals published several analyses concluding that decline in casual, multipartner sex had been the major factor in Uganda's earlier success against HIV.[11]

After many months of persuasion and consensus-building by especially Daniel Halperin, *The Lancet* printed a consensus statement late in 2004, recommending the ABC model for populations with generalized epidemics, emphasizing fidelity and delay for people not at immediate risk for HIV.[12] This statement had come from my colleagues and me, but they now included leading HIV researchers such as Helene Gayle (a former head of the CDC), Ward Cates (the president of Family Health International), and because of his own findings in the ABC study, Doug Kirby. More than 140 experts from thirty-six countries around the world endorsed the statement, including leading representatives of organizations like UNAIDS, WHO, the World Bank, the Global Fund, the United Nations Population Fund (UNFPA), the United Nations Development Programme (UNDP), the Alan Guttmacher Institute, Population Action International, and PSI. The heads of HIV/AIDS programs in several countries (including Ethiopia, India, Jamaica, and Uganda) and many other leaders (such as Desmond Tutu, Stephen Lewis, and President Museveni) also endorsed the consensus statement.

The statement included these revolutionary statements:

- *On fidelity:* "When targeting sexually active adults, the first priority should be to promote mutual fidelity."
- *On partner reduction:* "Partner reduction is of central epidemiological importance in achieving large-scale HIV incidence reduction."
- *On polarization:* "The time has come to leave behind divisive polarisation and to move forward together in designing and implementing evidence-based prevention programs."

In our most important statement, we agreed that condoms should be the primary strategy *only* for people at chronic high risk for HIV, such as prostitutes. But of course sex workers are a sliver of all populations. For "most people," we all agreed, the primary strategy should be *fidelity*, with condoms as a backup. That is, fidelity was the heart of prevention.

It might appear that we had won, but in fact the battle had only begun.

Ignoring the Rules

The statements from the top hadn't penetrated. In December 2002, the same month USAID did its about-face on fidelity, I had traveled with Claude Allen's delegation to Uganda. There I witnessed a nearly two-hour slide slow, jointly presented by USAID and the CDC on "What Happened in Uganda." It made no mention of fidelity, or even partner reduction and the decline of casual sex. It focused exclusively on latex, drugs, and vaccine research, as if these had caused the Uganda decline. I would see exactly the same presentation with the Tommy Thompson group in 2003. The intermediaries were shaping how the upstairs viewed the downstairs.

In fact, in 2002 the USAID mission in Uganda had recently funded a major condom policy and strategy document, and it called for placement of a salaried condom officer in each of Uganda's forty-plus districts. Fidelity had nothing remotely equivalent. I spoke out about this and was formally asked by the Uganda AIDS Commission (UAC) to develop a comparable strategy for fidelity and delay of debut. I went to Uganda to work with a low-level group trying to develop such a document, to complement the condom report. USAID refused to pay for any part of it. After I left, unfortunately the UAC was "advised" by donors to table our document. The mission in Uganda seemed determined to erase the elements that had made this nation stand out for so long as the only AIDS success story in Africa.

In 2004 I returned to Uganda and saw that still no donor—including USAID—seemed to be funding fidelity or delay of sexual debut, or any approach other than latex, testing, and drugs. Yet condom promotion was thriving. Of course, there was that pesky new ABC policy in USAID and PEPFAR, and a congressional earmark that a third of prevention funds had to be spent on "abstinence" programs. But, I thought then, perhaps the condom industry need not fear. I learned there that all fidelity and delay proposals had to go through the CORE Initiative global project of USAID. This was bad news for Africans because the CORE Initiative seemed merely lukewarm, if not actually hostile, toward fidelity-delay. I know that the leadership of a major CORE partner had been one of the strongest opponents of the ABC model, writing letters denouncing it to the heads of UNAIDS, the Global Fund, NIH, the Gates Foundation, and others. Despite the formal allotment of funds for ABC, no one was willing to act and ABC wasn't funded. Uganda's program remained broken.

The Yes! Project

In the summer of 2004, Africare asked if I would evaluate some AIDS prevention projects run by youth groups in Malawi, South Africa, and Zambia. Africare is like CARE International, but it focuses on Africa and most of the staff are either African-American or African. I had worked with three of these guys before, and I liked them all. I thought it might be good to get away from the firing line and back into the field for a few weeks. I'm always happier when I'm working in Africa or some other part of the developing world.

At the time the best-known and certainly best-funded program in South Africa was a youth project called LoveLife, begun in 1999. According to its Web site, "LoveLife is a comprehensive, evidence-based approach to youth behaviour change that implements, on an unprecedented scale, the international experience of the past twenty years—combining well-established public health techniques with innovative marketing approaches to promote healthy AIDS-free living among South African teenagers."[13] In fact, though, the program contained all the worst features of an American model forced on Africans. The approach is "sex-positive," assumes all or most teens are having sex, and focuses heavily on condoms. There is—or at least *was* at that time—a wink and a nod toward delaying sexual debut. As in: *Sure, great, but now let's get real: they are all doing it.*

As usual, the best survey evidence was ignored. A major, expensive national study called the Nelson Mandela Study found that 55 percent of South African youth said they'd had no sexual partner in the past twelve months.[14] It also found that "only one quarter of youth 15–17 are sexually active" and that 23.1 percent of youth ages fifteen to twenty-four reported abstinence after loss of virginity, or "secondary abstinence," in the past year. I mention this because the prevailing belief was—and probably still is—that once teens have their first taste of sex, there is no turning back. These findings challenge that view. If you are wondering what the summary and conclusions were for this study, perhaps you can guess: The Mandela survey made eleven recommendations about prevention. Every one related to condoms, drugs, and testing. I mean, why bother to do these expensive studies?

In addition to this survey, in 2002, LoveLife commissioned its *own* study to ignore: the First South African National Youth Risk Behavior Survey. It found that only 41 percent of the sample had ever had sex. The percentage reporting sexual debut before age fourteen was 14 percent. In contrast, there was the Yes! Project, which seemed sensibly designed. It sought out existing youth organizations in remote, rural areas and asked whether they'd like to add AIDS prevention to their activities. If so, and if they met other criteria, members received training in such income-generating activities as beekeeping, chicken raising, and seed oil pressing. Their programs could thus be financially sustainable. They were less reliant on AIDS World.

When I got to the field (with my wife Suzie as my unpaid assistant), I found the Yes! Project did indeed seem self-sufficient, and although it received some funding from the Gates Foundation, it largely steered its own course. In fact, the project was so low-cost that none of the youth groups had even gotten formal training in AIDS prevention. As a result, they'd fallen back on common sense and carried out AIDS prevention in a way they knew would be locally acceptable. The Yes! programs targeted youth with messages about delaying sexual debut and not having multiple partners. Members of participating youth groups typically went to villages and acted out little dramas to teach lessons about AIDS. For example, they might show a schoolgirl being tempted by a lecherous, civil servant-ish sugar daddy, and depict her good sense in refusing him. In fact, in both their content and methods, the Yes! programs resembled Uganda's efforts in the early years. Condoms were promoted, but their use was not a primary strategy.

Aside from the trickle of funding, there were two reasons the Yes! youth groups in Malawi, South Africa, and Zambia did not focus primarily on condoms. First, they were operating in remote rural areas, where condoms were not always available. As Museveni had observed in the speech that got him blacklisted from global AIDS conferences: "The practical questions of getting a constant supply of condoms may never be resolved." Second, many rural parents would not have let their daughters participate if condom distribution were the main activity—and Africare policy called for gender balance in all its projects. In fact, it was hard to enlist teens and young women early in the project, until the program "trustees" (local community supporters) explained that it actually promoted delay of sexual debut and fidelity. As I said in my report: "The single most important finding from this evaluation was that there is a viable model of AIDS prevention that seems replicable elsewhere in Africa and beyond. The model is low-cost, low-tech, culturally appropriate, sustainable, and to a great extent non-dependent on outside technical assistance or commodities, except for condom supply (and condom use is not the only behavior promoted)."[15] All in all, the Yes! Project is a good example of how less foreign direction is more, at least in African AIDS.

Africare was very pleased with my evaluation; they wanted me to present my findings to Bill Gates Sr., who had taken a special interest in this project. Alas, I came down with the flu just before I was to fly to Washington, D.C., to present, but I was well enough to put together a slide presentation that hit all the key points. My friend Clarence Hall gave the presentation to Gates Sr., and I knew Clarence would hit the highlights as I would have, without concern for political correctness. I have noticed that both Africans and African-Americans are usually nonresistant to the idea of fidelity and delay of sex, recognizing a phenomenon that could greatly help us in the fight against HIV.

Enter Templeton Support

I was in a remote part of Zambia when I got an e-mail from the John Templeton Foundation (JTF). I had never heard of these folks, but the assistant to a vice president informed me that her boss might want to support my work and ask when he could come to Harvard to meet and talk to me. I would later find out that a great many hopeful researchers bring all kinds of ideas and schemes to JTF, but only rarely does JTF take the initiative to contact a prospective grantee. Anyway, I didn't think much about it. When the appointed day arrived, Dr. Charles Harper arrived in my office. He turned out to be an Oxford-educated astrophysicist who had once been on the Harvard faculty. He told me he very much liked my book *Rethinking AIDS Prevention*, but wondered if I were possibly struggling along in an unfriendly world without much financial and moral support.

How could he have guessed? I told Dr. Harper that I was indeed struggling along, and I recounted the story of my removal from the USAID ABC study. In fact, with that grant income gone, it could be just months before I'd lose my position at Harvard. The School of Public Health, like no doubt many other parts of the university, expects faculty members to bring in their own grant money from the outside. Chuck helped me come up with a plan. JTF would support a small team to work with me. I quickly pointed out that I hated administrative work. Not to worry: JTF would hire an administrator. The plan called for me to be helped by a senior epidemiologist who had the quantitative skills I lacked, two doctoral students, and the administrator. JTF would even provide a nearly instant "bridge grant" to keep me solvent at Harvard while I put together a proposal and JTF responded.

For various reasons, most having to do with my own ambivalence about this responsibility, I did not finally accept the grant until September 2006. Then I hired Daniel Halperin as the epidemiologist (he was mostly an anthropologist, but he had postdoctoral training in epidemiology in public health), Allison Herling (later to become Allison Ruark), Timothy Mah, a Harvard doctoral student, and an administrator. We would become a powerful force. Daniel stayed on at Harvard after the project ended in April 2010, Tim Mah got his Ph.D. and almost immediately took Daniel's previous position at USAID/Washington, and Allison and I coauthored, among other things, my recent book *AIDS, Behavior, and Culture*.[16]

Meanwhile, the original director of the Center for Population and Development Studies became victim of a Larry Summers shakeup. He'd ended up being a supporter who was always willing to listen to me on AIDS and other issues. But now our center was put under another center and its director. That man told me candidly that a number of powerful people at Harvard would like to see me gone, and soon. I would have to prove empirically that fidelity and delay were important in AIDS prevention or my continuation at Harvard was in jeopardy. He had eminent professors like anthropologist Paul Farmer telling him that the only way to really prevent AIDS was to eliminate poverty, racism, sexism, and other inequities, and fidelity had nothing to do with it. So why didn't I conduct a randomized controlled trial (RCT) to prove what I was saying?

Well, RCTs take a minimum of three to four years and cost at least four million to five million dollars, especially if we expected to have "biological outcomes," or endpoints measured in decreases in HIV incidence. Yet our project was originally two and a half years and two million dollars. We were asked to do the impossible. How ironic. Harvard and the AIDS Establishment in general wanted to hold me to a standard to which it did not hold the well-funded industry. For example, there had been no RCT showing that increases in condom use led to lower HIV infection rates. Certainly no one had shown that less poverty or sexism led to lower HIV rates. Our small team had a much greater burden of proof. Why?

Another irony: The proposed randomized controlled trial could never have gotten funding anyway. Because it involved one group using condoms and another group *not* using them, it would be considered "unethical." The closest study of this kind was probably the "uncontrolled" one from 1995 in which Johns Hopkins researchers found the so-called Zenilman Anomaly. They divided a group of Baltimore-area men into three types of condom users—always, sometimes, and never—and followed them over a period of years examining differences in STD rates. Lo and behold, there were no differences among the three groups! This finding generated a flurry of letters to the editor, some quite agitated, and considerable debate. Most people decided that subjects had lied about their condom use, because after all we already *knew* condoms were effective, right?

JTF was actually willing to put an additional $2 million into a project whereby we would put out RFPs (requests for proposals) and African researchers would send us proposals, after which we would select and fund the best among them. But that was not to happen.

Meanwhile, as I stood on my teetering ledge at Harvard, blowback was growing in the wider world.

CHAPTER 10

Policy by Applause

In August 2006, Bill Gates addressed the Global AIDS Conference in Toronto. When he stated that the ABC approach (abstain, be faithful, or use a condom) had saved many lives, he was almost booed off the stage. Gates seemed surprised by the vitriolic crowd reaction. He conferred with someone, then returned to the microphone and proceeded to criticize fidelity and delay of sexual debut as nice but unrealistic ideas—and this time he got a sustained standing ovation. Razor wire and guards with rifles still surrounded the castle of AIDS errors. The forces keeping policy in place included the threat and reality of career damage, publication bias, and literal cheers and howls. Along with the UNAIDS "evidence-informed" approach to the epidemic, there was an applause-based one. Global AIDS policy seemed based on—or closely coordinated with—subjects audiences at AIDS conferences reacted to with enthusiastic applause and cheers (condoms, gay rights, more money for AIDS) or with catcalls (abstinence, fidelity, not enough money for AIDS, the fact that other diseases needed funding).

Policy by applause has several things *not* going for it. It represents neither science nor democracy. Special interest groups predominated at AIDS conferences, and these groups were giving the thumbs up or down to billion-dollar AIDS policies and programs. Powerful people like Bill Gates wound up changing their minds and favoring strategies that, at best, treated damage while the fire spread—with their own funding. This Gates incident was hardly a fluke. Here are a few others:

BANGKOK

In 2004, after the passage of PEPFAR (the African relief program), I attended the Global AIDS Conference in Bangkok, where I contended with the director of Planned Parenthood International in the "ABC vs. CNN Debate" (the latter referred to "condoms, needles, and negotiation," but in fact it was "condoms, needles, and condoms," because "negotiation" here meant negotiating condom use). During the Q&A period a delegate from Brazil stood up and proudly announced into the roving microphone, "Brazil will *never* accept an ABC program! NEVER!" The applause was deafening and sustained. Randy Tobias fared even worse. As the U.S. global AIDS coordinator, he had to endure ten minutes of angry shouting before he could begin to speak. In 2004 the United States had spent $2.4 billion on the epidemic, nearly twice as much as all other governments combined, yet Tobias attracted the abuse. These hecklers spared representatives from Japan and South Korea, which contribute minimally to the cause.

Ugandan President Museveni, invited to a key AIDS conference for the first time since 1991, also attended the gathering in Bangkok. A government official traveling with him told me that I had "empowered" Museveni through my writings to stand up for Uganda's original approach and his own role in slashing HIV rates. In his speech at the conference he again tried to explain how Uganda had used fidelity and delay of sexual debut to bring down HIV rates. The audience and the international press mocked him, however, and his speech spurred much anti-ABC publicity. Indeed, my colleagues told me afterward that the Uganda AIDS Commission (UAC) and the Uganda Ministry of Health, largely funded by the U.S. government, grew even more reluctant to support fidelity, for fear of offending the donors. Knowing how poor and needy Ugandans and indeed most Africans are, I cannot blame them for playing the AIDS game the way the donors and funders demand. Far less excusable is the hypocrisy of foreign AIDS experts who act innocent and insist they are just doing what the Ugandans ask them to do.

WASHINGTON, D.C.

In 2004 the former U.S. Surgeon General David Satcher organized a conference in Washington, D.C. There, I gave a forty-minute slide lecture showing how Uganda had brought down HIV prevalence by two-thirds, by following the ABC program. After the lecture, there was muted, polite clapping. A few minutes later, a female college student came to the microphone and exclaimed, "I think people should be able to have as much sex as they want, with as many people as they want!" You could almost imagine the comedian John Belushi stoutly delivering this line in *Animal House*. Yet here it got a thunderous standing ovation. Declarations like this one—sex first, AIDS second—sometimes leave me wondering if I'm hearing things. But there was an explanation, of sorts. A number of professional sexologists were on the panel and in the crowd, and many of the rest of the audience worked in the AIDS industry.

ETHIOPIA

In 2005, I gave the keynote presentation on AIDS prevention at the annual PEPFAR meeting, held in Addis Ababa. I presented what I thought was pretty thorough evidence that traditional AIDS prevention wasn't preventing anything at all, and that Uganda had shown that behavior change was both feasible and highly effective. After the presentation I looked out at a sea of upset, angry, offended, or blank faces. Not long after some tepid applause, a woman took the microphone and gave voice to the feelings in the auditorium: "We *all know* that condoms are the best weapon we have in our war against AIDS." This brought the crowd to their feet for loud and sustained applause. And these were not your everyday sexologists. They were the very officials running PEPFAR programs in Africa and around the world—the ones supposed to be carrying out fidelity programs according to U.S. law.

I remembered thinking that day in Addis that I had had dinner with some of these folks, our kids had played together, and we had sung old rock-and-roll songs together at parties. It's good to remind myself of this on a regular basis. These are good people who somehow have become terribly misled about AIDS prevention.

The Myth (or Exaggeration) of Disempowered African Women

On September 6, 2006, I testified before the House subcommittee probing the effectiveness of the ABC approach in Africa. Rep. Barbara Lee (D-CA) was seeking to repeal the 33 percent earmark and she knuckle-rapped me: "The rest of the world *gets it*." Her evidence for "rest of the world" was the Toronto conference she had attended that booed Bill Gates. I turned out to be the only one on the panel arguing for the Ugandan model of prevention. Because of my own politics, it pains me to report how my fellow liberals reinforced a variety of harmful, ethnocentric myths about AIDS in Africa in their testimony.

The first myth is that of the disempowered African woman. The CEO of CARE International, one of the world's largest private aid agencies, Helene Gayle, was one of the witnesses that day. She was a coauthor of our consensus statement. But on this date, Gayle said fidelity and abstinence might be fine, but we needed a "comprehensive" approach, meaning one that empowers women. As she put it: "We have a lot of examples from countries that have high rates of rape and sexual exploitation where girls report that they feel compelled to exchange sex for food. So clearly a message that focuses on abstinence and being faithful misses the point of the circumstances of these women and their lives." So let's now turn the microscope on the gender equality argument. It addresses three overlapping issues: violence, empowerment, and marriage.

VIOLENCE

Helene Gayle was expressing a widespread belief in the public-health community that violence fuels HIV infection through high-risk sex (including coerced sex and rape). Such pressures, it is believed, keep women from protecting themselves with condoms, counseling, and testing. So when the idea of behavior change arises, this response often comes back like a whipcrack: "*You* may have control over *your* behavior. How nice for you! But poor women of color don't have your advantages." There is no doubt that women globally, including in Africa, have experienced a nauseating wave of violence. But let's probe further to see what's really going on.

Gender equality advocates point to such studies as one in Soweto, South Africa, that found a clear correlation between HIV infection and intimate partner violence among women at a prenatal clinic.[1] Some 55 percent of them reported a history of physical or sexual abuse from a male partner, and physical violence correlated with HIV infection—although intriguingly sexual violence did not. The researchers posited that abusive men were more apt to be HIV-positive and to force risky sex on their women. However, the real world is not so simple. The study revealed a constellation of other factors that correlated with such hazardous practices as having multiple partners and selling sex. Here are a few of these factors: sexual assault while a child, forced first intercourse, and sexual assault as an adult by a nonpartner. In other words, sexual abuse rose and fell with riskier behaviors, which rose and fell with the chance of HIV, and all of these behaviors rose and fell with intimate violence. Note too that some of the abuse occurred in childhood and thus represents a somewhat different problem than gender equality.

This same study also investigated transactional sex (that is, for cash or other valuables) and found that it correlated significantly

with both HIV infection and violence. Transactional sex also correlated with intimate partner violence, substance abuse, and socioeconomic disadvantage. The researchers noted broader implications
for women's health, stating: "Abused women are also more likely to
suffer from depression, PTSD and other psychiatric problems, and
may abuse alcohol or other substances, using transactional sex to
sustain this habit. . . . Abused women in South Africa talk about
the experience of abuse changing the way they view relationships,
reducing their ability to trust men or expose themselves emotionally to men, and enhancing perceptions that a woman should get
something tangible from relationships."[2] Hence transactional sex
seemed more appealing to them than to other women, and of course
it boosts the chance of HIV. None of these findings about the complicated links between abuse and vulnerability, risk behaviors, and
HIV are surprising.

Other studies have failed to find *any* positive relationship between
intimate violence and HIV. In 2005, WHO researchers surveyed
twenty-four thousand women in ten countries and discovered that
between 15 percent and 71 percent of ever-partnered women said
they had suffered physical or sexual violence from an intimate partner. This study included data from four sites and three countries in
Africa: Ethiopia (rural), Tanzania (urban and rural), and Namibia
(urban). Here the study found just the opposite of Helene Gayle's
assertion: the more assaults, the less infection. In Namibia HIV prevalence was high (15.1 percent among urban women), while intimate
violence was lower than at any of the other African sites. Ethiopia
had the most violence (58.6 percent among rural women) yet the
least HIV prevalence (0.6 percent). Even within Tanzania, where we
had data from urban and rural populations, this inverse correlation
held.[3] This suggests there are far more important factors to HIV risk
than violence or the threat of it. Of course this study highlights the
danger of confusing correlation with causation, for otherwise one
might conclude that wife-beating prevented HIV.

Clearly, we should examine the relationship between violence and HIV more deeply. For example, people in long-term, stable partnerships have the lowest rate of HIV (and condom use), and promiscuity plainly increases the threat of HIV. These facts suggest that violent relationships are briefer and less stable, and presumably partners with less commitment to each other have greater chance of HIV. Why do women enter such liaisons, and how can they end or sidestep them? The bottom line is that it's complex. Causation isn't linear, but weblike.

EMPOWERMENT

Empowerment is the larger gender equality issue. Its appeal to Western women is clear. They have often fought key empowerment battles themselves, and they relate to African women who enjoy far fewer opportunities. The problem is vivid in Westerners' minds. They *understand* it. They have the tools to fight it in the West, and they can throw themselves into the battle in Africa. The more helpless African women seem, of course, the more urgently they need Western activists to come to the rescue. They become passive victims who can't aid themselves without powerful Planners riding to the rescue. Yet African women usually have considerably more power and control than well-meaning Westerners detect, in part because their options may not resemble those American women can point to in their own lives. Moreover, just because some people, like abuse victims, have much less power than, say, Americans, it does not follow that African women in general are helpless, reactive, and ruled by patriarchs and raging male hormones, and that we must attempt technology-based social engineering to save them.

Take this example: I knew a Swazi couple very well (the husband was my research associate). His wife found out he was cheating with an ongoing girlfriend. The wife said, "You can't go on having sex with me and her, especially with AIDS everywhere." When the husband refused to give up his new lover, the wife stopped sleeping with him. A couple of years went by. The husband's girlfriend ultimately died of AIDS, and the husband found out he was infected and he died too. His widow was terrified that she had HIV as well, so she got a test. She found she was clean. She had cut off sex with him in time. Wives are not powerless.

Insisting on empowerment first may actually disempower African women. For instance, a 2003 national survey in South Africa found that only a single-digit fraction of the population knew that having multiple sex partners puts one at risk for HIV infection. So we need better prevention messages, ones people can internalize and use. A message like "stick to one partner" is advice that individuals can follow, one that empowers individuals to save their own lives. But if the messages become weighted down with "what we *really* need to do is eliminate gender disparities or create employment opportunities," we're telling potential victims something else: "Eliminate inequalities and create jobs!" An individual is helpless to do this. Thus the social reform approach shifts the focus away from behavior people can change to vague, structural aspects of society that they can't. This ultimately disempowers women and men alike.

In 2007 my wife and I spent two weeks in Senegal and The Gambia. In this little corner of West Africa, as in most Muslim countries, HIV rates are very low. Women also have less freedom, power, and ability to "move about" (as they say euphemistically in Africa) than in countries like Swaziland, South Africa, and Botswana, and they have few secret or not-so-secret lovers. However, Senegal is known for its pattern of migratory women from the rural interior to the trading centers of Dakar and the coastal towns. It is women who predominate in trade, not men, but they belong to various formal associations. Social control mechanisms keep a rather strict eye on them and their behavior when away from home.

While interviewing throughout Senegal and in parts of The Gambia, I could not get rid of the nagging thought that if somehow Islamic and social controls weakened and these women became more empowered, more of them would have extramarital partners and HIV infection rates would rise. More freedom means more freedom to sleep around. So the impact of greater gender equity on HIV infection rates is not straightforward. Female empowerment, although crucial for so many reasons (including better health outcomes for them and their children), may have an AIDS-related downside. In fact, greater women's emancipation repeatedly correlates with higher HIV rates. Women are freer in Kampala than in the low-HIV countryside. They are freer in high-HIV Botswana and South Africa than in low-HIV Somalia and Ethiopia. They are freer in the top fifth of wealth than in the bottom, and have three to four times the HIV rate. They are freer with primary or secondary education than without— and have twice the infection rate.[4]

These facts don't mean we abandon gender equality as a goal. They mean we stop thinking about it as a prerequisite for curbing AIDS.

MARRIAGE

Overlapping with the issues of violence and empowerment, marriage is the third leg in the gender equality argument. A deadly variant of the powerless woman myth arose around 2004 (although an early version appeared in a CDC/Uganda report in 2003): marriage is hazardous for African females. Columnist Nicholas Kristof gave voice to it in a *New York Times* piece warning against both abstinence and marriage: "What kills young women is often not promiscuity, but marriage. . . . Indeed, just about the deadliest thing a woman in southern Africa can do is get married."[5] In other words, it's safer to be a prostitute than an African wife.

As a UNAIDS publication put it: "It will be important to raise popular awareness about the risks marriage poses to teenage girls, and encourage families to try to *delay marriage for as long as possible.*"[6] Why stay single? Here is the standard industry reasoning: Women can say no to sex if they're unmarried. Women can't if they're married. Therefore, married women are at more risk than unmarried women. It's a neat, simple formula, but its lethal fallacies are worth stressing again. This reasoning ignores three facts:

- Married women always have a lower HIV prevalence than unmarried women (single, divorced, widowed). For instance, the 2004–05 Demographic and Health Survey found that HIV prevalence among married women was 6.3 percent, far lower than infection rates among widowed (31.4 percent) or divorced (13.9 percent) Ugandans.[7] We see the same pattern everywhere: better to be married than not married when it comes to AIDS or STDs.
- Wives frequently infect husbands, which follows from the fact that young women have much higher infection rates than young men in Africa.
- African women have more agency than their well-meaning defenders in the West suppose (as shown for instance by the frequency of Ugandan wives leaving unfaithful husbands).

My colleagues and I gave a press conference in Uganda in December 2006. I noticed a well-known condom advocate in the audience, waiting to pounce during the Q&A portion. And so she did: Why, she demanded, do we support fidelity even though African men routinely cheat on their wives? I answered, "If men cheat on their wives, surely that is the behavior we want to change." No response to that. There never is. I said the same thing to Rep. Barbara Lee (D-CA) when she asked me about male straying: "If faithless men are infecting their wives, it's the men's behavior that needs to change, and that's fidelity." She switched the topic: "But what about women and the access to condoms?"

No one can admit that they get it, that we've put sexual freedom before protecting women. In fact, I doubt the anti–behavior change activists have really thought through the implications of their position. If asked, they probably couldn't tell you why sexual freedom trumps fidelity, why they must forever hold the position that changing sexual behavior = bad, condoms = good. Yet this ridiculous, dangerous myth persists. Stephen Lewis, the UN secretary general's special envoy for HIV/AIDS in Africa, repeated it, citing information from UNAIDS: "Marriage can be dangerous to women's health. . . . There is virtually no defense against that reality: the power imbalance in marriage is too great to permit or to request the regular use of condoms. Thus it is that the classic 'ABC' intervention doesn't work in the one place where the risk for the woman may be greatest."[8]

> To impose a dogma-driven policy that is fundamentally flawed is doing damage to Africa.[9]

> A distortion of the preventive apparatus is resulting in great damage and undoubtedly will cause significant numbers of infections which should never have occurred.[10]

Those aren't my words. They are Stephen Lewis's. He would be right—if he were speaking generally. But he was referring to low condom usage in Uganda.

The Myth of African Promiscuity

Beneath the myth about marriage harming women's health is the myth about African promiscuity. Sometime after my testimony at the earmark hearing, I heard Rep. Chris Shays (R-CT) say that "asking an African to abstain is like trying to repeal the law of gravity." I regularly see my colleagues—liberals who swear they despise racism—use near-racist stereotypes of African male sexual behavior. A highly respected anthropologist friend of mine recently informed me that "someone did a study" and found that "African men have no idea what *we* mean by faithfulness." In the global community that is AIDS World, one routinely encounters some variant of this sentiment: "Most Africans begin sex at an early age and then are highly sexually active, with many sexual partners." One can hear this idea from USAID, UNAIDS, the CDC, the World Bank, the Global Fund, UNICEF, and other organizations. I can't count the times Western AIDS experts have told me that "an African man's idea of fidelity is to be faithful to his current five (eight, ten . . .) girlfriends." When I've asked what percentage of African men have five or ten partners per year, I usually get no answer, or I'm told we can't believe surveys about sexual behavior because "everyone lies."

Where did the myth of African hypersexuality come from? From adventurers, first. The notion that African men routinely have ten or fifteen partners dates back to early missionaries and explorers like Sir Richard F. Burton, who fascinated Victorian audiences with lurid tales of sex in the jungle. This idea sold books. But the myth of promiscuity also stems from my own field of anthropology. In the colonial era, anthropologists studied African sexuality largely to emphasize how it differed from ours. From the outset they described it as "wild, animal-like, exotic, irrational and immoral." I have already mentioned the profound impact of Margaret Mead's depiction of unrestrained sex in Samoa. Early accounts almost amounted to ethnopornography, and it was sometimes difficult to distinguish anthropologists' tales from the explorers'. Leading anthropologists gave the world titles like *The Sexual Life of Savages* that soon became something of an embarrassment, as once-remote, tribal peoples became more urban and educated (sometimes earning Ph.D.s in anthropology, and studying *us*). A fear of being confused with ethnopornographers, or at least of seeming prurient, kept anthropologists away from sexual behavior from the 1950s till the early AIDS pandemic, some thirty years later.

Then a sudden urgency emerged for information on African sexuality. As anthropologist Quentin Gausset has pointed out, the scholarly lens turned again to the exotic. We heard about dry sex, injection of monkey blood into human pubes, wife sharing, circumcision and scarification rituals practiced on a large scale with the same knife, sugar daddies, and beliefs that sex with a virgin, even a baby, could cleanse one of AIDS. There were also reports of extremely high STD rates and of Africans having myriad sex partners, almost as many as those reported by "fast-track" gay men. Early in the African hyper-epidemic, scholarly papers appeared attributing it to promiscuity. Some relied on highly *non*representative victims, such as truck drivers, fishermen-traders, and sex workers. We must remember that no one really knew at that time why AIDS was ravaging Africa. It was probably natural to assume that because American AIDS seemed to strike gay men with vast numbers of partners, afflicted Africans must also have had a great many. And if truck drivers and sex workers had scores of them, probably most Africans had at least multiple partners. After all, polygyny thrives in Africa.

But these early studies gave a very distorted picture. As I told the subcommittee at the earmark hearing: "Only 23 percent of African men and 3 percent of African women reported multiple sex partners in the last year, according to the most recent DHS surveys. Among unmarried youth fifteen to twenty-four, only 41 percent of young men and 32 percent of young women in Africa reported premarital sex in the last year." Yet even today, documents on African countries typically assert that "most" youths are sexually active. The authors are "experts" in major donor and implementing organizations, people who should know the current research data. But they seem oblivious to it, in my opinion, and their claims are false.

Nowadays, *most* Ugandans ages fifteen through twenty-four do not report intercourse in the previous year, unless they are married. Now, we have to take all self-reported sexual behavior with a grain or two of salt. Women might underreport sex and men overreport it. The important point here is that our best survey data are greatly at odds with what white folks *believe* about African sexual behavior, and we have acted—and spent billions—on our beliefs and not our best empirical data.

The Myth That Poverty Drives AIDS in Africa

Dr. Lucy Nkya, a psychiatrist and a Tanzanian member of Parliament, had flown six thousand miles to attend the hearing. As if speaking for her continent, she asserted: "Coming all the way from Africa, I'd like to insist that AIDS is a disease of poverty." She added: "If you are poor, you are going to engage in behavior which is going to put you into risk of getting infected." Even female empowerment, she said, would fail "if we don't address the issue of poverty, especially among women. This is evidenced by a program I conducted in a brothel whereby I was able to empower those woman economically, and we managed to remove more than 67 percent of those women from prostitution."

I had worked with Dr. Nkya in these very Morogoro brothels to help these women just before my first trip to Uganda in 1993, and we have published articles together about the plight of women forced into prostitution. And, although she didn't say it, I know that Dr. Nkya works *mainly* with prostitutes. So her job doesn't require her to think much about females in the general population. *Of course* poverty is a major factor in driving women into sex work and *of course* they and their clients should use condoms. But, unfortunately, Dr. Nkya was represented as speaking for Africa's needs in the general AIDS domain, not in the infinitely smaller prostitution domain. She spoke of Africans' need for "life-skills training," the "vicious cycle of compounding poverty," and the need to provide a "holistic HIV/AIDS prevention package." She called for more and more condoms, and they had to be free. She used all the words expected of an industry guest from Africa. A holistic approach has come to mean "anything but altering sexual behavior."

Social reform was not the first approach to AIDS in Africa. But when remedies centered on individuals seemed ineffective, the Cultural Experts arrived. "Critical anthropologists" like Merrill Singer and Hans Baer and political economy–oriented anthropologists like

Paul Farmer and James Kim have focused on the links between disease and large social forces. They said: treat society, not just the person. Farmer proposed the crucial perspective for understanding AIDS was structural violence—meaning such societal "structures" as racism, sexism, and inequality that caused direct and indirect harm to people. Sexual risk-taking was just one more manifestation of social injustice. One could view health systems as mechanisms for "maintaining and reproducing the working class" and for "imperialist expansion and bourgeois cultural hegemony." Following this line of thought, the poor don't need condoms; they need money, power, and collective bargaining muscle. We have to overthrow exploitative systems and redress unfairness, and these goals take precedence over, for example, the ABC program. Until we do, condoms will suffice.

Let's consider Botswana. Seventy percent of it lies in the desolate Kalahari Desert, and in 1965, the year before independence, it was the third poorest country on the planet. Botswana had little infrastructure and widespread illiteracy, and it periodically suffered drought and famine. It was nowhere. But since independence, it has been a phenomenon. Its economy has grown faster than any other on earth, averaging 9 percent a year from 1966 to 1999. Its standard of living now approximates that of Turkey or Mexico, and the global organization Transparency International has called Botswana the least corrupt country in Africa.

Botswana's astonishing rise stems mainly from careful fiscal policy, but also from key Western values like tolerance and the rule of law. Here was the poster child for social reform theorists, an African society that had beaten back poverty, expanded citizens' rights, and in general successfully fulfilled the prescription. And do you know what happened? As Botswana prospered, leading public and private sector donors shoveled money into AIDS prevention, investing probably more per capita than any other developing nation. Western experts took the cash and gave us the world's second worst epidemic.

We see this elsewhere, of course. Other relatively affluent nations like South Africa and Swaziland also have high HIV rates, much higher than the poorest countries in Africa. If we look *within* nations, we see the same phenomenon: the more wealth (and usually education, which correlates with wealth), the more AIDS. We've known of this correlation since 1983, and I discussed it at length in *Rethinking AIDS Prevention*. In 2006 Roger England wrote in *The Lancet*: "Contrary to prevailing views, evidence from DHS's in Kenya and Tanzania indicates that poverty is not a risk factor for HIV."[11] After twenty-three years the fact remained "contrary to prevailing views." Poverty does contribute to other types of HIV epidemics outside Africa, as with the sex workers that Lucy Nkya mentioned. The problem is that African AIDS is so different from AIDS everywhere else that it is hard for us to imagine that higher income and education might be risk factors there. Of course, once again, if poverty mattered, we'd be in real trouble, because we have no idea how to end underdevelopment from the outside. The Botswanas and Taiwans of the world wrought their miracles from within.

The Myth That "Unprotected" Sex Drives African AIDS

Representative Shays, the subcommittee chair at the earmark hearing, had just returned from a trip to Africa that had been supported and/or hosted by Planned Parenthood, whose raison d'être is to get the maximum number of contraceptives out into the world. Shays interviewed a number of "representative Africans" the organization had arranged for him to meet, and as a result he felt "it would be an absolute outrage if someone *could* have had a condom and didn't because somehow they weren't available because we were diverting money in a different direction." He added that "to hear people describe using condoms more than once because they weren't available is pretty gross."

In my own testimony I explained that the more condoms we

export to Africa, the higher infection rates tend to climb. But it was hopeless. Representative Shays simply believed that condoms were the answer. He had seen—or had been shown—a slice of reality and believed it was the whole: poor Africans craved condoms and the Bush administration was cruelly denying them. Here before him my colleague Lucy Nkya was demanding more condoms. Shays seemed a thoughtful, well-meaning man, and he graciously said my testimony had "tremendous credibility," but he didn't seem to listen to it. He had already bought into the Great Abstinence Fantasy: that the choice is condoms or celibacy. It's a false dichotomy—uninfected, faithful couples can have all the passionate sex they want with zero risk of AIDS—and I am always surprised to see professionals fall for it. The real choice is between risk reduction and risk elimination. It's between Botswana and Uganda.

Condoms are just one strategy in risk reduction, but their failure exemplifies it. Indeed, no risk-reduction approach has *ever* cut back sexually transmitted HIV over broad populations in generalized epidemics. This statement holds true for treatment of STDs counseling and testing, diaphragm use (as an expensive research program supported by the Gates Foundation confirmed), microbicides, "safer sex" counseling, and income generation.[12] Yet we seem no closer to a vaccine today than we were twenty years ago. In fact, one of the most recent microbicides actually made HIV transmission a little easier.

I had an interesting exchange with Representative Lee about this issue. From the transcript:

> *Representative Lee:* All I'm saying is, why can't we just repeal the earmark and say to countries, develop whatever plan makes sense to address this terrible deadly disease. That's all I'm saying . . .

> *Dr. Green:* I agree with the intent of what you're saying, but I think in practice what happens is poor countries ask for the program that they know that there is money for.

Representative Lee: Oh, Dr. Green, come on. You know how you're sounding, very patronizing. Countries have the ability—and I've spent quite a bit of [time in] Africa . . .

Dr. Green: I lived there.

Representative Lee: Countries around the world have many unbelievable people who know how to address epidemics, pandemics, disease if only provided the resources and the support and the technical assistance. I can't believe that in any country at this point, if we didn't help develop and go in and do the things we need to do to support their efforts, that they couldn't be successful. So I can't buy the poor country notion.

Dr. Green: Again, I agree with your intent. I wish there was some way to let these countries choose for themselves without imposing our priorities on them.

Representative Lee: Well, I think we can.

By the end of the hearing, Representative Lee promised to work as hard as possible to defeat the 33 percent earmark for abstinence and fidelity. I commented that no one likes earmarks—that is, Congress forcing certain amounts of spending, seen as bullying by bureaucrats—but without requiring a fixed sum for behavior change, U.S. agencies would almost certainly revert to the old formula of condoms-drugs-testing. They wouldn't try to limit multiple and concurrent partners at all.

At this Helene Gayle said, in essence: Nonsense. There never was such an old formula. "I used to run USAID. We *never* promoted condoms only. Behavior change was always central to our policy." But she didn't say that they defined "behavior change" as *switching to condom use.* They actually measured behavior change in units of latex. It was still this way in 2006 for nearly all U.S. and other government agencies. I had no chance for further comment at the hearing; otherwise I would have explained that fidelity and sexual delay were merely rhetoric before the PEPFAR earmark. No real funds ever went to these programs globally.

There should be a Nobel Prize in public health, because advances like draining swamps have saved far more lives than medicine itself, as valuable as it is. If one existed, an award would surely go to Uganda. Politicians like Representative Lee would *have* to pay attention. We might keep healthy people from dying.

As I boarded a taxi and headed back toward my hotel, one of the author William Easterly's lines ran through my mind: "Compassion is driving the fight against AIDS in Africa in a direction that may cost more lives than it saves." The people I criticize throughout this book are for the most part sincere, motivated, and well-meaning. I am like them and they are like me. Yet they were ignoring solutions to the hyperepidemic. How could they?

The Confirmation Bias

What if there were a contest for the greatest obstacle to good thinking? What would you nominate? The psychologist Raymond Nickerson might cite the confirmation bias. This phenomenon alone, he has written, could "account for a significant fraction of the disputes, altercations, and misunderstandings that occur among individuals, groups, and nations."[13] We're all vulnerable to the confirmation bias—me, you, the people you love, Einstein, Nickerson himself, everyone. It's like our susceptibility to optical illusions. The best we can do is to take conscious steps to counter it. The worst we can do is to deny it and pretend the illusion is real. In essence, this bias reassures us that we're right. It's a near-invisible yes man in our heads that directs us toward evidence that supports us and away from evidence that doesn't. As a result, we unwittingly attend to and overemphasize facts that back our positions, while spurning or minimizing those that don't. Fair-minded individuals can thus skate over information that conflicts with their premises. You may make people listen, but you can't always make them hear.

Francis Bacon described the confirmation bias back in 1620. Once the mind forms an opinion, he observed, it pulls supporting evidence to it like a magnet, while setting aside contrary cases so its "conclusions may remain inviolate." He added that this mental quirk keeps superstitions like astrology alive, because "men, having a delight in such vanities, mark the events where they are fulfilled, but where they fail, although this happened much oftener, neglect and pass them by."[14] Consider Britain's decision to help invade Iraq. Tim Dowse, the former UK head of counterproliferation, said that the Foreign Office simply believed too strongly that Saddam Hussein had weapons of mass destruction. "We had got out of the habit of questioning ourselves and our assumptions," he admitted. "And that is something that we have certainly given a lot of attention since, to make sure it doesn't happen again."[15]

These are well-informed people, and one surprising fact about the confirmation bias is that knowledge tends to make it worse. Because we let in more supportive evidence than nonsupportive, the more we know overall, the more certain we may feel that we're right. As a result, we can get even deeper into the hole we have dug for ourselves. As social psychologists have shown, the stronger our commitment, the less likely we are to admit error. Fervent members of cults predicting doomsday—those who sell their houses and cars in anticipation of it—will watch the hour of annihilation come and go, and then cling even more strongly to the cult. This experience is called cognitive dissonance. We deem ourselves smart and sensible, and when we see evidence that contradicts this self-image, we rationalize it away. We don't want to feel like fools, so we end up as greater fools. This is the pitfall of arrogance, the "pride that goeth before the fall." Everyone makes mistakes, and the more clearly we see our own fallibility, the less fallible we become.

The confirmation bias has yet another aspect in matters like AIDS policy. The psychologist L. L. Thurstone caught the essence of it in 1924: "The more urgent the impulse, or the closer it comes to the maintenance of our own selves, the more difficult it becomes to be rational and intelligent."[16] Sexual freedom lies deep in people's psyches. It brings out strong emotions, bearing on love, privacy, lust, independence, and self-fulfillment. For some people, especially gays, it can affect their basic public identities and sense of self-worth. All these factors exaggerate the confirmation bias. For instance, they helped breed the evidence-informed approach of UNAIDS, an overt policy of stressing confirmatory evidence. They intensified the wrap-around pressures of ideology, in which group members share the same confirmation bias and help maintain it in each other. And they led to policy by applause.

You don't have to have cofounded a street gang to do good science—but it has benefits. Outsiders, often beyond the reigning ideologies, see the confirmation biases of the majority more clearly. Because everyone is vulnerable, we have to listen to contrary voices, people on the ground, thinkers with novel perspectives. We also need strong, deliberate, well-highlighted efforts to overcome the bias in public matters. We're all at risk for this thinking defect, and we have to keep searching for ways we might have erred. In Africa we could have started by opening our eyes.

CHAPTER 11

Cracking the Error Edifice

Remember that pro-fidelity statement in *The Lancet* signed by 150 professionals in 2004? The cover of the November 4–10, 2006, issue of *The Lancet* proclaimed: "It is less contentious to promote abstinence and faithfulness than sex education, condoms, and safe abortion, but these are what is needed." Two weeks later, the cover read: "The greatest challenge to sexual-health promotion in almost all countries comes from opposition from conservative forces to harm-education strategies." By "harm-education strategies," they clearly meant condoms and needles. Medical journals in general and AIDS journals in particular had made it an unwritten policy not to publish evidence that challenges the harm-reduction thinking of the established industry. I've noted many examples, but in light of the confirmation bias introduced in the last chapter, I want to explore the matter more fully.

When journals get wary, they can deploy several tactics. For instance, they may require twice as many peer reviewers as usual. I know of two articles—Norman Hearst and Sanny Chen's landmark UN study of condom effectiveness and an article of my own (with three coauthors from Harvard and Hearst from UCSF)—that had to go through six peer reviewers instead of the usual two or three before appearing in *Studies in Family Planning*, the journal of the Population Council. But at least they published the articles; Hearst and Chen had been rejected by at least one AIDS journal, and I have long since stopped counting my rejections.[1]

Journals may also send only a fraction of submissions on a topic out for review, and they may reject letters and commentary without explanation. Overall, they exercise the power to determine which interpretations reach the public and which don't. Consider the issue of African promiscuity. I submitted articles to several journals in which I showed that Africans had fewer sex partners over their life-times than Europeans or Americans. Indeed, the data were in plain sight in the DHS surveys. Yet editors or peer reviewers rejected all these articles, so years went by during which the AIDS community assumed that Africans had more sex partners than Westerners.

The Lancet rejected without explanation a commentary in which I discussed this matter. Then in 2007 it published a study that made exactly this point: Africans were less promiscuous, yet had much higher HIV rates.[2] How is this possible? The authors had come at the data from a completely different angle than I had. They criticized fidelity and delay of sexual debut, suggested marriage was a risk factor for HIV, praised condoms, implied that Uganda's success stemmed from its "strikingly" high levels of condom use, and provided a sidebar extolling Brazil's "adoption of sex positive approaches" (such as handing out condoms in schools) and Thai-land's "100 percent condom-use" program. The authors concluded: "The data make a powerful case for an intervention focus on the broader determinants of sexual health, such as poverty and mobility, but especially gender inequality." *The Lancet* published a study rein-forcing almost every myth that robs the taxpayer of money, pumps it into a bloated AIDS industry, and keeps Africans and others sick and dying. These mistakes buried the real implications of Africans' relative lack of promiscuity.

Jim Shelton ultimately published two commentaries exposing some of these errors in *The Lancet*, notably "Ten Myths and One

Truth about Generalised HIV Epidemics," but he had to talk about his decades-long "love affair with condoms" and present latex in the best light without violating science. And he wields some power at USAID.[3] And consider the case of John Richens at the University of London. He sent *The Lancet* an article about risk compensation in which he declared: "Massive increases in condom use worldwide have not translated into demonstrably improved HIV control in the great majority of countries where they have occurred."[4] None of the peer reviewers found any fact-based reason to reject it, yet *The Lancet* still refused to publish the article. Richens had to threaten a lawsuit to make the editors change their minds. *The Lancet*, to its credit, has retracted some articles in error. In February 2010, for example, it totally withdrew support from a 1998 article purporting to show that the mumps-measles-rubella vaccine helped cause autism. This pseudo-study had led many parents to shun the vaccine for their children and caused much needless suffering. But the consequences were trifling compared to those from African AIDS. Maybe one day this influential journal will retract its cover claim about this disease as well.

The Lancet is not alone, of course. The November 2006 cover of *Reproductive Health Matters* was a blank but tastefully decorated page with only four words: "Condom yes. 'Abstinence' no!" The editors devoted the whole issue to extolling condoms and trying to discredit behavior change unrelated to technology. Every contribution in that issue was "sex-positive," and it was understood that journal readers were hip and critics were prudes. Does abstinence mean not kissing, not touching? the editor wondered disingenuously. She went on to say, amazingly, that "condoms have no well-funded champions anywhere, not even a full-time person at UNAIDS." That was like saying the sun never shines on the Sahara. Almost everyone at USAID, UNAIDS, the World Bank, and all the other major donors have been devoted champions of condoms, and of course this editor's own taxpayer dollars were supporting a condom officer in each of Uganda's forty-plus districts. Condom champions are so ubiquitous that even the Bush administration seemed to fear the anticondom taint.

How easy has it been for condom supporters to get published? In November 2009 the journal *AIDS* let the contraceptive organization FHI edit an entire supplement. It surrendered its editorial function to this group. In the parable of the blind men and the elephant, each man touches a different part of the animal and describes it differently. "An elephant is like a large hose," says the one who feels the trunk. "It's like a tree," says one who encounters the leg. But in an ideology the blind men all crowd around a single part like the tail and declare: "An elephant is like a snake." There were times when I thought that the medical establishment would never understand that an elephant is not like a snake.

Nonetheless, as desperate, disease-wracked African nations began following the Uganda path, the fact pile continued to grow. Between my 2003 *Rethinking AIDS Prevention* and 2007, more and more evidence was reaching print about the real dynamic in Africa. Jim Shelton and a handful of others, almost always with Daniel Halperin urging them on and sometimes writing first drafts, began to publish important findings that challenged the entrenched paradigm. Because Jim was not Ted Green, because he had impeccable condom credentials (better than the ones I once had), and because he was always careful to declare his love of condoms, he managed to slip some very subversive papers past peer review. In addition, Daniel and his replacement at USAID in Washington, D.C., published an article about risk compensation, one I would refer reporters to during the Pope Benedict uproar in 2009.[5] And I (or was it my coauthors?) even managed to soften my own language enough to sneak a couple of articles through peer review in 2006.[6] For by then, even as *The Lancet* was emblazoning falsehoods on its cover and activists were publicly jeering Bill Gates and Randy Tobias, some truths were getting hard to deny.

Rwanda and the Overestimation of HIV

Like Uganda, Rwanda has seen horrors. The slaughter of up to one million Tutsi by their tribal rivals the Hutu in 1994 was the worst murder spree in recent times. Overall, most experts assumed that this staggering bloodshed and chaos would increase infidelity and promiscuity in Rwanda, and boost HIV prevalence. Yet the data strongly suggest the reality is—as usual—much more complicated. The 2006 Rwanda Demographic and Health Survey, the first to ask about HIV there, found a prevalence of 3 percent—half the rate in Uganda and much lower than earlier UNAIDS figures for Rwanda. This new information suggested that the proportion had never reached any level like 30 percent, as some researchers had initially estimated, nor even the 13 percent figure from the UN in 1998.

What had kept AIDS under control in Rwanda? There several factors at play. First, Rwandans typically delay sexual debut. Only about one in ten males and one in twenty-five females ages fifteen to twenty-four said they'd had premarital sex in the previous year. Fidelity was even more common. Among sexually active people ages fifteen to forty-nine, only one in twenty-five men and one in a hundred women reported multiple partners in the past year. These are exceptional figures. Condoms and circumcision played minor roles in keeping AIDS under control. Rwanda has one of the lowest rates of condom use in Africa, and male circumcision is relatively rare. In other words, if we ignore fidelity and delay, we can only wonder how this destitute nation torn apart by genocide could have so much less HIV than its neighbor Uganda.

In March 2006 I wrote an op-ed in Uganda's daily paper, *New Vision*, about the DHS findings next door. I did not submit it to an American newspaper (despite my earlier publications) because I felt certain of rejection. I observed that HIV rates throughout Africa were lower than we were hearing from the West. I wasn't guessing or extrapolating. The numbers came straight from the DHS: HIV was declining in Africa. Yet calling attention to this fact can get one in trouble. One can be accused of not caring about Africans, of being in denial about the severity of the epidemic, or, in extreme form, of denying the epidemic itself. So I was surprised to see a front-page article in the *Washington Post* a few weeks later called "How AIDS in Africa Was Overstated: Reliance on Data from Urban Prenatal Clinics Skewed Early Projections." The article detailed how HIV infection rates were considerably lower than previously estimated. The rates continue to drift downward, as an article in *The Lancet* recently showed, and as I have argued in *Rethinking AIDS Prevention.*[7]

This news, to the extent it has gotten out, has been greeted not with joy and relief, as one might expect, but with skepticism and disbelief. As I pointed out in my 2003 book, it suits the fund-raising and political agendas of some international AIDS players to minimize or deny evidence of falling HIV prevalence, to highlight fiery worst-case scenarios, and to exaggerate the rates. They even describe viral Armageddons and rationalize these fear appeals by saying, "We can't rest on our laurels. Infection rates may begin to rise again." However, officials have also told me privately that news of even slow improvement might cause donors to shift funds elsewhere.

Beyond Uganda

Other changes were occurring in 2006. Journals were publishing evidence that HIV prevalence was starting to decline elsewhere. After Uganda, Kenya and Zimbabwe were the first two countries to exhibit a falloff. Moreover, a growing handful of us noticed that we regularly saw changes in sexual behavior along with prevalence decline, as in the widely circulated (but perhaps unpublished) figure below (see figure 1). In 2005, UNAIDS issued a study that evaluated a variety of different data sources and concluded that HIV prevalence had fallen in Zimbabwe over the previous five years. The study stated that reductions in rates of sexual partner change—that is,

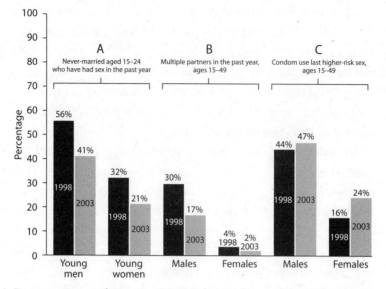

Figure 1   Kenya: Changes in "ABC" indicators between the 1998 and 2003 Demographic and Health Surveys (DHS). *Source*: DHS data 1998–2003.

greater approximations of fidelity—contributed to the improvement.[8] It also credited high rates of condom use with nonregular partners, although these rates were already high by 1999. As former AIDS ambassador Mark Dybul observed about this nation: "Perhaps one of the most interesting things is that the greatest behavior change was in abstinence and fidelity. The relative change in condom use was not as remarkable."[9] Not mentioned is the fact that we know most of the condom users are *inconsistent* users, and that studies in Uganda (and elsewhere) have clearly shown that inconsistent condom use does not protect against HIV infection in the long run (for example, over a year of intercourse).

An analysis of several countries sought to determine through mathematical modeling whether the drops in prevalence were tied to changes in sexual behavior or simply stemmed from death. The study concluded that in Uganda, parts of Kenya, Zimbabwe, and urban

Haiti, "HIV prevalence has declined further than would be expected through the effects of mortality alone." These improvements have been attributed to changed sexual behavior.[10] Other studies found that fidelity seemed to be the sexual behavior change with the most impact on prevalence rates.[11] The fact that Zimbabwe and Haiti are leaders in *decline* of HIV in their respective regions is further evidence that AIDS in Africa (and certain areas outside of the country) is not really about poverty. Certainly HIV decline is not related to good governance! In fact, there seems to be no case yet where HIV prevalence has fallen in Africa without prior declines in multipartner sex and in premarital sex. That is, the correlation so far is 100 percent, while the correlation with condoms is, if anything, negative.

Finally, some news of these developments was reaching the journals. But restrictions remained. I had written *Rethinking AIDS Prevention* as a book to get around them, and soon three other critics of AIDS World also turned to full-length books: Jim Chin, Helen Epstein, and Elizabeth Pisani.

Triple Hammer

As mentioned, I first met Jim Chin on an AIDS evaluation team in the Philippines in 2000. In a briefing with the health and population officer at USAID/Manila, our group heard the usual dire visions of AIDS fanning out to engulf the Philippines. I said I disagreed with this assessment.

"Are you serious?" one of the briefers asked me.

"Absolutely," I said. "I don't think the Philippines will ever have a serious epidemic—unless boys stop getting circumcised and sexual behavior makes a radical turn toward multipartner sex."

After the briefing, Jim introduced himself and said, "I'm glad I won't be locking horns with at least one member of our team." I already knew him a bit by reputation. His public comments flew in the face of the pronouncements of UNAIDS that AIDS was getting worse everywhere, therefore please send more money immediately. Other team members recalled the endless discussions between Jim and me on that consulting gig. Sometimes we'd be driving in a van together for hours, and the two of us would talk nonstop. They said it was fascinating to hear two guys whose thinking was so original and contrary. It says something that no one ever asked us to shut up, to give it a rest.

At the time we met, and over the years to follow, Jim was growing more and more marginalized, being passed over on the invitation lists for conferences and evaluation teams, because he openly mocked the party line that AIDS was threatening to engulf the world. Finding himself in circumstances not unlike my own, Jim finally had to write a book to expose parts of the AIDS racket most obvious in Asia. He and I have been and remain allies on his main issues from the start. I have turned to him often for advice on Asian epidemics, and I quoted many of his then-unpublished ideas and observations in *Rethinking AIDS Prevention*, material that later appeared in his 2007 book, *The AIDS Pandemic: The Intersection of Epidemiology and Political Correctness.* Yet Jim's focus is primarily Asia, so he never quite agreed with me on the futility of condoms in Africa or on the importance of fidelity and male circumcision.

In his book he assailed the propaganda that AIDS was getting worse and worse, so we needed to keep pouring more money down the ever-widening throats of PEPFAR, UNAIDS, the Global Fund, and similar organizations. Here is Jim's basic argument: Like any other contagious disease, HIV spreads according to how many total people the average sick person infects over his or her lifetime. When, on average, an infected person infects more than one other person, we say an "epidemic spread" will result. When, on average, such a person infects fewer than one other person, epidemic spread will not occur. It's a simple but powerful concept. Almost everywhere except in the African hyperepidemics, the average infected person infects fewer than one person at the national level. We see a pattern of miniepidemics only among high-risk groups such as gay men, prostitutes, and injecting drugs users—always small minorities of any national population. As Jim showed, even if they infect their immediate sex partners, the virus does not usually spread further into the population because most wider societies lack the same patterns of partner mixing and exchange. Thus instead of HIV "bridging to general populations," as many AIDS specialists have long assumed and predicted, we find what Jim bluntly calls "bridges to nowhere." The explosions of HIV warned about in countries like China, India, Indonesia, and Russia simply never happened, the experts notwithstanding.

It was a critical argument, and for some AIDS activists this line of reasoning was tantamount to Holocaust denial. But I have long agreed with Chin, and events have proved him right. As we've seen, HIV rates are slowly declining throughout the world (except for the United States), before any "bridge to gen pops" occurred.

Helen Epstein's engaging *The Invisible Cure: Why We Are Losing the Fight Against AIDS in Africa* (2007) took the reader on her journey of discovery about African AIDS.[12] The book highlighted the danger of concurrent partnerships, while offering a mild, almost incidental criticism of condom programs. Epstein also took shots at abstinence and the involvement of faith-based organizations, stances that may have helped acceptance of her book by some of the same colleagues who were furious with me.

Before 2003, Helen believed the solution lay in sanitizing "transactional" and commercial sex, increasing condom use, and improving "social conditions that make people vulnerable to HIV infection in the first place . . . including poverty, unemployment, and discrimination against women."[13] In early 2002, I brought her into an informal group of independent, contrarian thinkers who engaged in passionate and robust e-mail discussions about the enigmas of global and especially African AIDS. That same year Helen started publishing articles saying that Western solutions had not worked in Africa, and that we needed to address the main driver—multiple concurrent partners—with interventions of fidelity and partner reduction. In *The Invisible Cure* she took aim at myths about African sexual behavior, especially that early sex is common and multipartner sex is the norm. She focused on concurrent partners as the missing explanation for Africa's hyperepidemics, and she termed networks the "super highway of infections" and casual sex the "on-ramps" feeding into the traffic.

Elizabeth Pisani, who had served at UNAIDS from 1996 to 2005, was the third barrel in this shotgun of truth. How can you dislike a book called *The Wisdom of Whores: Bureaucracies, Brothels, and the Business of AIDS*? Her sassy title no doubt shocked conservatives, and many liberals sensed betrayal in calling AIDS a business. Yet this charming, disarming book earns the 2008 Edward Green Award for Whistle-Blowing in Science—and for good reason. Both an epidemiologist and journalist, Pisani has published with such well-known AIDS experts as Michel Careal, Marie Laga, and Bernard Schwartlander. She has solid insider credentials. Indeed, I referred to her earlier, mainstream writings several times in my *Rethinking AIDS Prevention*.

The Wisdom of Whores tore the roof off UNAIDS. Pisani made it clear that Diogenes would have had a near-endless trek through its halls, even passing her by. The AIDS Mafia—her term—presented its numbers to the world "in their worst light," she observes, and did so consciously. By exaggerating the danger, UNAIDS scared wealthy nations into donating more and more funds to AIDS (while claiming such fear appeals couldn't work in Africa, among the people actually threatened with death). Their fabrications have led to calls to shut UNAIDS down. Pisani tells us that UNAIDS head Peter Piot staffed the agency with "mavericks" who worked in the "real world." As a result, the "sober WHO lifers with whom we shared our corridors must have been startled by UNAIDS staff with nose rings and Jean-Paul Gaultier shirts." She herself got caught up in the exciting, crusade-like atmosphere she found at UNAIDS, at least in the mid-1990s. Of course, even if someone starts off as a maverick, the freedom cage can descend—especially once he or she holds privileged positions in a multibillion dollar initiative. Pisani notes that over time "UNocracy" would wear the real mavericks down, and "they would either get out or sell out."[14]

Pisani's book reveals how UNAIDS became first and foremost an ideologically driven advocacy agency—and ultimately a fundraiser with a huge gravitational field. "Two things were getting in the way—ideology and money," she writes. "In the AIDS industry, we have too much of both." The ideologies of AIDS activists "influence what we do about sex and drugs and determine how we do it. Money, of course, follows the dominant ideologies." They had at first thought money would make it easier to prevent a wider epidemic; in the end, they found that it just gave them more to spend on favored causes. En route to its huge flow of cash, UNAIDS became a major source of bundling. Pisani quotes a disgusted friend at the World Bank, who told her: "The UN institutions are professional beggars, and beggars go where the money is. So you get 'culture and AIDS,' 'kids and AIDS,' 'fish and AIDS.' I'm just waiting for 'climate change and AIDS.' "[15]

Pisani also exposes the notion that HIV epidemics had great potential to spread into general populations. As early as the late 1990s, scientists and others at UNAIDS knew HIV was not going to storm through the wider world, she says (Jim Chin and I had realized this earlier). How then could UNAIDS frighten the wealthy nations into coughing up billions of dollars to address HIV? They had at least three ideas: economy, babies, and innocent wives.

THE ECONOMY

First, they said, think of all the money we can save by addressing AIDS early, forestalling epidemics that were sure to erupt even in parts of the world where UNAIDS mischief makers knew they would not. How much cheaper to provide a condom or a clean needle today (these are Pisani's examples) than to spend thousands of dollars caring for an AIDS patient ten years from now? To support this argument, explains Pisani, infection rates had to be alarming and getting worse exponentially. Thus UNAIDS director Peter Piot warned in 2000 that India could be at the brink of a swift-moving epidemic of Ugandan proportions relative to society. In other words, some 150 million people might soon have HIV. Yet India's national AIDS program, NACO, had been disputing UN statistics as early as 1994, when it officially questioned the basis on which UNAIDS calculated that it then had 1.75 million people with HIV. NACO also claimed exaggeration of the 2000 statistics, and NACO director Prasada Rao explained: "There is no basis for these projections and the UNAIDS headquarters in Geneva could not explain how they reached these estimates."[16]

Similarly, UNAIDS announced to the world that there was the "potential for an explosion" of AIDS in the Philippines and sought to flood the nation with condoms. Yet in this conservative, Catholic country condoms were unpopular and people had relatively few sex partners. As UNAIDS itself admitted, the prevalence of AIDS never exceeded an extremely low 0.01 percent, and an article in the *New York Times* observed that in these islands "a very low rate of condom use and a very low rate of HIV infection seem to be going hand in hand."[17] There was never any chance of an HIV "explosion" here, as Jim Chin and I and our whole team wrote in 2001.[18]

One trick was to wave the red flag of growth rate, as if it indicated severity. Here's how it worked: Suppose a country has a very low incidence, say, a hundred new cases annually. If it rises to two hundred, you can say AIDS is doubling every year—even if the second hundred cases resulted largely from better diagnosis. Still, it sounds pretty bad, like the disease is out of control. UNAIDS liked to trot out China for this ploy. It has 1.3 billion people, so imagine how destructive the epidemic would be in ten years. If it became another Botswana, a quarter of a billion people would be HIV-positive, almost as many as the entire population of the United States. In the same way Indonesia, the Philippines, Russia, and Ukraine all became figures of fear— yet none has epidemic potential outside of small, high-risk groups. As Pisani says, we should be "deeply suspicious when we encounter phrases like 'one of the world's fastest growing epidemics.' It's the first sign of a beat-up"—a deliberately misleading exaggeration.

BABIES

The second way that UNAIDS frightened wealthy nations into contributing more money to address HIV was babies. The organization asked us to think of the poor babies infected at birth. These helpless infants couldn't possibly have done anything wrong. What chance did they have? What's more, these babies faced the likelihood of joining the exponentially rising number of AIDS orphans. As we've seen, the image of suffering babies had first caught President Bush's attention, which led to PEPFAR.

INNOCENT WIVES

The third sleight-of-hand Pisani describes of her colleagues—and even herself, she is honest enough to admit—was to highlight the image of innocent wives who are being infected by wayward husbands. First the wives get the virus and then, she wrote, "we implied HIV would blaze though the general population." Of course, as Chin pointed out earlier, HIV dead-ends unless a majority of wives have outside concurrent sex partners. It turned out that UNAIDS already knew that this almost never happened. A hyperepidemic requires that a substantial minority of women, as well as men, have concurrent sex partners.

UNAIDS had authority and people heeded it. But it did not simply present false data to the world. Pisani is straightforward about the political machinations of her mafia: "We imitated Big Tobacco as best we could, packaging up the data for different politicians, lobbying various interest groups, massaging the media."[19] So when UNAIDS staffers saw politicians like Representative Lee repeat their arguments, arguing passionately for the need to end gender inequality and poverty, they knew these honorable people were purveying falsehoods they themselves had bred, spread, and lobbied for. But they felt the end justified the means. After all, how else would governments cough up cash for "deviant outcasts" like hookers, transvestites, junkies, and gays? Here's how: use wide-eyed babies and violated wives as bait and you can bundle AIDS with women's emancipation, sexual liberation, and poverty eradication too.

If the end was to stop AIDS, however, this approach was the most egregious backfire in the history of public health, wasting billions of tax dollars and shouldering aside low-cost, low-tech, community-based, culturally grounded strategies like Uganda's that had saved millions of lives. Ultimately, these deceptions worked because the feedback loop never included the supposed beneficiaries. Donors want to know they have done good and recipients want to keep the money river flowing, so there is little incentive to report what actually matters on the ground. "If you torture the statistics enough, they'll confess to anything," Pisani wrote. "Doing honest analysis that would lead to programme improvement is a glorious way to be hated by just about everybody."[20]

For years UNAIDS said that the AIDS problem was growing worse all over the globe. Yet unending bad news would not succeed as a fundraiser indefinitely. "I found myself trying to walk the tightrope between 'it just gets worse and worse' and 'we know how to stop this thing,'" Pisani explains. There had to be some good news or donors would give up. She wrote a UNAIDS report about Senegal, Thailand, and Uganda, the developing countries where UNAIDS had detected improvement. Regarding Senegal, she even tiptoed into heresy, mentioning as one of several factors: "Sexual activity begins relatively late and extramarital sex is relatively limited." Pisani recalls "sitting in Geneva banging the HIV-is-coming-to-get-you tom-toms" until by 2007, global AIDS spending had risen to ten billion dollars annually in developing countries alone.[21]

But a tower of pretense can't stand forever. By 2007 there were too many random sample, population-based sero-surveys (that is, surveys of blood, not just interviewees) showing HIV prevalence figures considerably lower than the UN estimates. The United Nations finally had to restate its figures and also mention that, oh by the way, HIV prevalence has actually been declining for quite a few years. UNAIDS quietly added this admission to its Web site around November 2007. It was too late to prevent the Institute of Medicine from stating authoritatively in its official assessment of the fifteen-billion-dollar PEPFAR program that "the rate of new HIV infections continues to grow."[22] How misled was the IOM? In 2009, UNAIDS admitted that the spread of AIDS had peaked *thirteen years before*, in 1996, when about 3.5 million new infections occurred, and that in 2008 the number of new HIV infections was roughly 30 percent lower. Pisani was perhaps too close to UNAIDS and Asia to fully grasp the implications of her remarkable revelations on Africa, the sheer life destruction to which UNAIDS falsehoods have led. Describing the day she quit, she concluded: "In the AIDS industry, I felt we were all whores."

CHAPTER 12

Chasing the Wild Programs

In October 2007, Norman Hearst and I were in Uganda, just a week or two before the release of its latest National Strategic Plan (NSP) for HIV. When it appeared, we were not too surprised by the contents. It proved the logical endpoint of donor philosophy, because it virtually gutted the parts that had saved lives. Indeed, this draft plan could have come straight from any of the southern African countries, where AIDS has spiraled out of control. It was a basket of medical "services" already proven (through randomized controlled trials and/or consistent associational studies) *not* to work in generalized epidemics. Fidelity was absent from the key numerical goals and targets that would presumably guide policy for the next five years. It all came riding in on the well-decorated float of human rights.

Hearst and I tried to stop it. We called attention to this travesty at the Uganda offices of USAID and PEPFAR. These people seemed vaguely alarmed—not by the tentative plan, but by the prospect of two American health professionals causing trouble. The United States funds 85 percent of all HIV/AIDS programs in Uganda, yet we heard innocent-sounding statements like: "Oh well, this is a Ugandan process and who are we to interfere with what they want?" However, Hearst and I had just interviewed many Ugandans supposedly involved in developing the plan, including the two cochairs of the NSP Prevention Committee, Sam Okware and Rev. Sam Ruteikara.

Both men were shocked to learn that language and impact indica-tors—the benchmarks for measuring achievement—for both fidel-ity and abstinence had vanished from the NSP. They had worked to include them through a formal participatory process with various local stakeholders. As Rev. Sam would later write in the *Washington Post:* "We promoted fidelity for sexually active people, abstinence for young people, and condoms only as a last resort. . . . Repeatedly, foreign advisors erased our recommendations. When the document draft was published, fidelity and abstinence were missing."[1] In fact, every Ugandan we spoke to wanted behavior change in, not out, of the plan. Every one of these officials said they believed fidelity and delay should be central to AIDS prevention in their country.

What was going on? Some AIDS bureaucrats told us that the omission of behavior change was a mere oversight that would soon be corrected. Of course, the repeated erasures suggest the opposite: censorship. Indeed, this particular "oversight" has occurred with odd frequency over the years. I have been hearing the excuse since at least 2003, when the head of the Uganda AIDS Commission first uttered it to me. Despite Hearst's and my efforts, we failed. The "targets and indicators" in the final October 2007 document had come straight from Geneva, from a UNAIDS consultant whom few Ugandans have ever met. There were also stirring passages about empowerment, achieving gender equality, and defeating poverty. Remarkably, these goals did not find their way into the indicators, although you'd expect to see them if the author thought they were effective at reducing HIV.

The Uganda approach therefore became the Botswana–South Africa–Everywhere approach. Ironically, the comparable Strategic Framework for Botswana (2003–2009) took its cue from Uganda in the good old days. One of its stated goals was: "Promote education on 'Zero Grazing' or abstinence." Meanwhile, a suspicious statistic blaming most HIV infections on marriage had also appeared. In his *Washington Post* op-ed, Rev. Sam wrote: "The plan states that the HIV infection rate among married couples is 42 percent, twice as high as the rate among prostitutes. Our requests for the source of this statistic were repeatedly ignored."[2]

In this same document we read that the rate of new infections was rising in Uganda, that an HIV incidence of 0.2 percent to 2.0 percent exists, depending on the part of the country. There were 132,500 new cases in 2005, including 25,000 transmitted from mother to child. "The stagnant and worsening HIV trends in Uganda actually date from about 2002," the final report observes. "There is a strong possibility that the negative HIV trends are at least partially attributable to phasing out of 'zero grazing' and other partner reduction/fidelity-focused campaigns of the late 1980s."[3] I had to rub my eyes and look again. The author in his Geneva office had apparently realized that fidelity worked, yet kept cutting it out of the Strategic Plan. What could he have been thinking? What motivated him to eliminate a cheap, effective anti-AIDS strategy, knowing that men and women would die because of it? *Maybe ideology kept him from acting*, I thought. *Maybe fear of stigma had silenced him.*

Norman and I weren't done. We complained in private to the highest levels of PEPFAR that we, America, were complicit in hijacking Uganda's program, scorning the clear will of the cochairs of the Prevention Committee and many other Ugandans we had consulted. Hearst and I also drafted an op-ed when we returned to the United States. Several years earlier World Vision's vice president for Africa, Wilfred May, and I had written in the *Washington Post*: "American partisans must not be allowed to make decisions from thousands of miles away—and from a culture even more distant—on ways African couples protect themselves from this most intimate of diseases."[4] Now Hearst and I were prepared to say it again, with Uganda as the example under threat.

Yet we thought we had better first notify Mark Dybul, the AIDS ambassador at the Office of the U.S. Global AIDS Coordinator (OGAC), because he and his deputy supported evidence-based AIDS prevention. We did not want our op-ed to cause them embarrassment. They reacted quickly and asked us not to publish it. In return, OGAC would lean on its local U.S. government people in Uganda. In addition, we would gain seats on the newly formed Technical Working Group to ensure that removal of fidelity and delay indicators did not occur elsewhere in PEPFAR, in the hyperepidemics. So Hearst and I held our fire. The U.S. mission in Uganda came up with an "annex" that contained some program targets and measures related to fidelity and other sexual behavior. Of course, an "annex" has a tacked-on, subsidiary feel to it and USAID and the CDC might easily forget about it in the years—maybe weeks—to come. Despite this, Hearst and I accepted the proposal.

As this book went to press, the Strategic Plan through 2012 contains none of the changes apparently promised to Ambassador Dybul: no fidelity or partner reduction. Condoms and testing dominate it. Dybul was gone too. Hillary Clinton had fired him during her first few days as secretary of state, probably because of his support for the ABC model.[5]

Warm-up to Reauthorization

PEPFAR was a five-year program, and as it drew to a close, the U.S. government sought fact-finding statements to guide it forward. Most important, it asked the Institute of Medicine (IOM) to evaluate PEPFAR accomplishments and the Government Accounting Office (GAO) to report on the effectiveness of the "abstinence" earmark. The IOM report appeared on March 30, 2007. We've seen how UNAIDS misled the IOM about the trend of HIV infections. Yet its findings disturbed me in other ways, enough that, when asked, I submitted a dissenting opinion to Congress. (I was asked to testify, but I was unable to because I was hosting a conference in South Africa on the hearing date. Norman Hearst testified, however, and it may have been better for Congress to hear from someone other than me.) In my dissent I pointed out that, among its other shortcomings, the IOM report seemed to assume that abstinence or even abstinence and fidelity together were mere distractions from effective strategies, such as condoms. It often mischaracterized Uganda's ABC approach or showed it in a negative or false light. For example, the report said: "It is important to understand that ABC represents neither a program nor a strategy, but a goal of changing key behaviors."[6] Of course, why would anyone fund a goal with no program or strategy? It would be like funding "good will" or "niceness." The money would have no place to go.

The report also went after the usual straw man: abstinence-only: "The Committee has been unable to find evidence for the position that abstinence can stand alone or that 33 percent is the appropriate allocation for such activities even within integrated programs." Hadn't they read the legislation? It unequivocally stated that abstinence would *not* stand alone. The document further urged that we "put the accent on preventive measures of proven efficacy on a much larger scale."[7] "Proven efficacy" did not seem to refer to fidelity or delay, although in the seven or eight African countries where prevalence first declined, we always see significant partner reduction beforehand. Again, the report authors seemed unfamiliar with this literature. At times I wondered if some malevolent gnome held the keys to these studies and barred people like these committee members from seeing them. But of course the research was easily available for download on the Internet and copying in the library.

As a member of the Presidential Advisory Council on HIV/AIDS (PACHA), I helped write an internal document, a white paper on PEPFAR, that we hoped would influence the design of PEPFAR II— or "PEPFARther," as we were calling it. New people had joined PACHA since my term had begun and maybe I was just lucky, but they all seemed reasonable. We reached consensus and finalized the document in October 2007, just as my term was ending. It was much more evidence-based than the IOM report, and it came from a body with "presidential" in its name. Hearst and I also came to Washington, D.C., in September 2007 to brief the House Foreign Affairs Committee on the science behind a comprehensive approach to AIDS in Africa that emphasized behavior change. We provided documentation with recent high-level, peer-reviewed articles. In late 2007 this committee asked the GAO to "come up with a formula" for dumping the "abstinence" earmark. Suddenly the GAO had to inaugurate a process that seemed fair and objective to cut the successful African AIDS strategies.

The GAO was not new to this controversy. In 2005 its members went on a guided tour of a few African countries and on their return, armed with "field research," they came down on the side of "letting local government agencies decide" how to prevent AIDS in a particular country. The GAO emissaries had spoken almost entirely to health and population officers from USAID, PEPFAR, and the CDC, people with long backgrounds in contraceptive promotion. They had talked to the foreign-aid superstructure that supplies money and bends local decision making. It was the too-familiar failure to truly listen to opinions outside the AIDS industry.

In January 2008 the GAO phoned and asked to interview me. They had a list of questions to send me about PEPFAR and the earmarks in particular. Hearst was on their list of interviewees as well—we suspected that we would be the only ones to break the consensus and tell the GAO to emphasize behavior change. But at least they would hear two voices instead of just one. If my responses were in writing, documentary evidence would exist that the GAO had heard the truth about African AIDS, for future historians who will no doubt find much of interest in the handling of this holocaust. I remember seeing this question on the GAO form: "What are the strengths and limitations of the 33 percent requirement for abstinence until marriage programs?"

Hadn't *anyone* read the bill? The GAO had mischaracterized the very earmark it was supposed to investigate. I explained that the 33 percent was for delay *and* fidelity. "And even though there is a great deal of skepticism in the West about abstinence," I wrote, "this is the main behavior we find in unmarried Africans, ages fifteen to twenty-four. However, it becomes rare after age cohort twenty to twenty-four, and it has been found empirically that the B of ABC prevention ('being faithful,' or reduction in number of sex partners), is the single most important behavior accounting for the rise and fall of HIV incidence and prevalence." Moreover, as I noted about Uganda, the title of its new Strategic Plan was *Moving Toward Universal Access*, which meant access to technology, because people already have universal access to fidelity. "The emphasis on behavior change has all but disappeared in this Plan," I wrote. "Uganda now conforms to what donors and especially entrenched implementers like to fund and implement. In the view of a growing number of us, this Plan may be good for business but not for public health."

PEPFAR II

When the bill came out of the Foreign Affairs Committee, it eliminated the requirement that 33 percent of prevention funds go to fidelity and delay. Instead, it directed the global AIDS coordinator to promote a "balanced" prevention program country-by-country, including every element of ABC. In the end, after all the congressional hearings, testimony from people on both sides of the issue, and from the GAO interviews, the new legislation authorized forty-eight billion dollars over five years for AIDS, malaria, and tuberculosis, and thirty-nine billion dollars for AIDS itself. It doubled the annual donation to the Global Fund, up to two billion dollars.

The bill also added significant new language. It said that efforts to promote fidelity, abstinence, delay, partner reduction, and condom use "represent important elements of strategies to prevent the transmission of HIV/AIDS." It ordained that AIDS strategy promote abstinence from sexual activity and encourage monogamy and faithfulness, and encourage "the delay of sexual debut and the reduction of multiple concurrent sexual partners," among a list of approaches. Critically, the bill required that at least 50 percent of AIDS prevention funds focus on fidelity and delay. Furthermore, the global AIDS coordinator Eric Goosby had to base the 50 percent allocation to fidelity-delay on objective evidence. If he found any reason to provide less than 50 percent for any country, he had to report the reasons to Congress within thirty days. So the amount for prevention was unstated, left to the coordinator's discretion on a case-by-case basis, but because objective evidence does not exist for condoms in southern Africa, presumably condoms should not receive more funding than fidelity and delay.

After all the promises to dump behavior change requirements of any sort, I was happy to see pragmatism prevail—and I was rather surprised at this outcome.

Churning Hormones

Overall, by 2008 so much evidence had appeared that the challenge was to assimilate it. On March 10 of that year, Dan Rather interviewed me for a TV broadcast, along with Stephen Lewis, the recently retired AIDS ambassador for UNAIDS. I was amazed to hear Lewis utter the following rationale for the condom approach in Africa: "In the United States, more than 50 percent of teenagers are sexually active by the age of eighteen. Why should it be different in other countries?" One wonders why the U.S. taxpayer spends countless millions of dollars to obtain detailed data on the sexual behavior of Africans if officials are not going to cite that data? In this case it's probably because a strong majority of Africans ages fifteen to nineteen in fact do abstain unless they are married. Women marry early in a number of African countries, so a significant amount of female teen sex is actually marital sex.

But Lewis went on to smile slyly and confide in Rather, guy-to-guy: "Hormones are churning in Africa! So why the devil would you insist upon abstinence when you *know* people are sexually active! If you want to protect them, you gotta use a condom."[8] Ambassador Lewis had access to Demographic and Health Survey statistics showing that most sexually active adults, married or not, report having only one partner in the previous year. In 2006 this figure was 93 percent in Uganda, and 89 percent in Zambia. He also had data available from Kenya, Zimbabwe, and Ethiopia, as well as Chin's and Epstein's books, which can hardly have escaped his attention. This "churning hormones" thinking is pure racial stereotyping and justification for a shoulder-shrugging, behavior-is-hardwired, condoms-focused approach. Yet the data are clear: more condom use is associated with more casual and commercial sex and often higher—not lower—HIV infection rates. If you want to protect them, you gotta use something other than a condom.

CHAPTER 13

A Bridge to Somewhere?

Condoms remained as ineffective by 2010 as they were in 1994 or 2001 or 2007. Indeed, the high-quality studies still show that none of the Western-conceived "best practices" have ever had any effect on generalized epidemics.[1] Regarding prevention, we would probably have done better leaving Africa alone. Has the Western approach— supported by falsehoods, appeals to high morality, cash, and a carrot- and-stick ideology—changed significantly? The answer is complex. Meanwhile, the days of easy money have, if not vanished, been cut back. The Great Recession has severely cut funds for life-preserving antiretrovirals (ARVs), and we may soon see another tide of death.

Botswana: Back to a Future

In Botswana, home to the world's second worst AIDS epidemic, the bitter failures of business-as-usual had clearly sunk in by December 2007. In that month Botswana officials asked me to make a presenta- tion to its full Parliament. I had several in-depth discussions with the minister of health and other key figures, as well as the secretary of education and former president Quett Masire. I was happy to find that these officials wanted to change course and focus on fidelity and male circumcision, as well as discouraging cross-generational sex and early sexual debut. They now wanted to do AIDS prevention much as they probably would have done if Western experts and money had never materialized.

Botswana is now the first African country I've seen where a majority of the key players—including UNAIDS and WHO—seemed on board with evidence-based prevention, as early as 2007 and 2008. I saw the government did not have to fight the UN organizations or the PEPFAR representative. I found that several key people had read my *Rethinking AIDS Prevention* and were actually . . . well, fans! What a change. I was asked to provide advice to the Botswana National AIDS Committee, for the prevention component of the National Strategic Plan. The change was apparent in former Botswana president Festus Mogae. He had been one of the AIDS industry's best friends during his presidency. He listened to the UN, PEPFAR, Merck, and Harvard and followed their advice. Who can blame him? He made Botswana the first country in Africa to provide free ARV drugs for anyone who tested HIV-positive and got publicly tested for HIV himself, to counter the stigma of taking the test. Yet HIV rates soared.

Festus Mogae is still so dedicated to AIDS prevention that he attended the 2008 International AIDS Conference in Mexico City. There, when an interviewer asked him what steps Botswana was taking to combat HIV, he said: "One is to try to bring about a delayed debut of sexual activity by young people both male and female. . . . The other is a reduction in the number of concurrent sexual partners." He did not mention condoms. In early 2009, Botswana broke the chain and launched a national fidelity or partner reduction program called Break the Chain. The program name was referring to networks, of course, but I couldn't help sensing a deeper meaning.

Sayonara to Harvard

At Harvard my program, the AIDS Prevention Research Project, had operated out of the same Victorian wood-frame house from which the university expelled 1960s "turn on, tune in, drop out" guru Timothy Leary. We worked on the fringe in general, although we seemed the only ones in the entire university who seemed to be focused on AIDS prevention. When a Harvard-wide one-day conference on African AIDS prevention took place in early 2008, and the organizers had somehow failed to notify us, it was as if our merry band of freethinkers had tuned in and dropped out itself. Harvard professors are better known for advocating "free drugs for the poor," a highly popular program on all campuses. It saves lives and offers the moral satisfaction of shaming powerful drug companies into cooperation, so students find it highly appealing. Students find cutting the number of sex partners highly unappealing. I would have too, back in my licentious, polyamorous days.

The widely admired anthropologist Paul Farmer is a leading proponent of reform. He is an outstanding and decent man, and I respect him for his passionate dedication to his cause. In a written debate on AIDS prevention, he had the courage to say he agreed with me on the basics.[2] His main criticism of one essay I wrote was that I did not emphasize the need to overcome poverty and restructure power relationships. I sympathize, of course, but inequality and poverty don't worsen African AIDS (and we can thank our stars for that). We don't have to transform society to save lives and, as the experience in Botswana showed, greater wealth doesn't help in the AIDS arena. Farmer once wrote: "Anthropology, the most radically contextualizing of the social sciences, is well suited to meeting these analytic challenges [of African AIDS], but we will not succeed by merely 'filling in the cultural blanks' left over by epidemiologists, physicians, scientists, and policy makers."[3] I completely agree. We anthropologists look at the big picture and traditionally have not hesitated to point out unfair power relationships. Yet here we can further contextualize the analysis by filling in blanks not just in the culture, but beyond its periphery. When a vast AIDS industry imposes profit-generating formulas from the outside, discrediting cheap but effective methods, this context becomes the essence.

By February 2008 a new director was in charge at the Population Center. She was a sociologist and because a fellow behavioral scientist should better appreciate the role of behavior change in AIDS prevention, we hoped our program would expand. Yet at our first formal meeting, the director informed me that my program did not fit her vision of where the Center should be headed, nor with what others are doing in the AIDS field at Harvard. She said she wanted to limit center activities to "large randomized controlled trials" (RCTs) and "working with large data sets" and doing "advanced statistical analysis." I reminded her that we lacked the time and funds to do an RCT, and it would almost certainly be considered unethical, therefore undoable, anyway: imagine proposing to withhold condoms or the option of monogamy in a control group! I pointed out that our work was original, groundbreaking, policy-impacting, paradigm-challenging—in fact, it seemed to be the only AIDS prevention program anywhere at Harvard.

She replied that she had "thought and thought in order to try to find some place" where our project might fit in with her new plans, but alas she couldn't. At any rate the decision had already been made. In an unguarded moment, the director later told a member of our team that our work was "journalism, not science." Sometimes I wonder if the truth about AIDS prevention will likewise burn up unnoticed, high above our bustling world, like Leary's ashes. They were launched on April 21, 1997, by NASA in a Pegasus rocket and remained in orbit for six years until the rocket burnt up in the atmosphere. However, the rest of the world was disagreeing more and more with her—not just in Congress, but in other surprising places.

Into the Old Fibworks

In May 2008, as our program was ending at Harvard, I was asked to join a new UN global steering committee called "AIDS 2031—The Programmatic Response." Michel Sidibé of Mali, then the deputy director of UNAIDS, had set it up to get UNAIDS to "really think outside the box" and reshape AIDS prevention in light of "recent" findings. The committee was also to plan AIDS prevention strategies for the future, in ways that are "more sustainable, and that address the points raised by some of our fiercest critics." I think I heard my name echoing about in that last phrase.

At first I thought the invitation was a joke. But there seemed to be a business-class ticket to Geneva in my name. So in May 2008, I flew to Switzerland, and there Michel told me to my surprise that he had read *Rethinking AIDS Prevention* and had become a supporter and admirer. He had run UNICEF's Uganda program in the 1980s and early 1990s and had taken part in initiatives to delay sexual debut. He pointed out that much of what I had said in my 2003 book had since come to pass—or had been confirmed by even more evidence. Michel turned out to be the main—and perhaps only—person behind bringing me onto this steering committee.

At the first meeting, we started off going around the table and, being the important people that we were, we each made what amounted to an opening statement. I explained that generalized epidemics differ crucially from concentrated ones and therefore compel us to address multiple concurrent partners. I spoke for four to five minutes and made this point in several ways, in case it was missed. But when the woman appointed to register the points discussed at the meeting read them aloud, my points were not there. Of course that's how the confirmation bias works: Inconvenient evidence gets swept out of sight. AIDS World had been acting this way for a long time. But things improved later in the afternoon. Michel and some other key, respected figures said in public that they agreed either with partner reduction or with building our interventions upon indigenous knowledge, leadership, and organizations.

That evening, we all went out to eat. I loathe three-hour dinners, a trait that has been in my family for at least three generations, so it may have a chromosomal basis. At this Thai restaurant we were still on our third or fourth *starter* dish almost two hours into the affair.

Once a few prominent minds had had a little beer over dinner, they slid back into the old thinking. *In vino veritas*, indeed, but also *in vino non veritas*. Here's what I heard:

- What we really need is *protected sex*. It's just a matter of making condom use *consistent*. Fidelity can't work because African men *always* cheat on their wives and African women can't resist men or even expect decent treatment from them.
- If African governments could only *choose how they do AIDS prevention*, they would quickly torpedo abstinence (and by implication, fidelity and delay). It's been proved that the real risk factor in Uganda these days is *marriage!*

I could see why Michel had invited me to participate.[4] The committee faced other problems, which UNAIDS and all African AIDS organizations will have to address. First, it had mingled concentrated and generalized epidemics together in the discussion, so people often misled each other. For example, an African colleague might say that we need to find culturally appropriate ways to reduce partnerships and someone else would respond: "The real problem is, we are not implementing programs where the virus is actually found—among despised, sometimes illegal, social outcast groups." But that's where the bug lurks in concentrated epidemics, not in Africa—it's everywhere but especially among better educated and wealthier people.

The second program the committee had to face was the Dry Zambezi Problem: using genuine feedback. My colleague Vinand Nantulya told the group that we had to mobilize local communities, that their representatives actually had to sit at this very table and speak for themselves. The chair quickly agreed: "Oh, yes, we need to engage civil society." Vinand replied that he didn't mean "the usual suspects." "Civil society" refers to people in NGOs or community-based organizations that we have created with our AIDS billions or that follow the party line to gain our funding. Vinand was referring to the true leaders at the local level: chiefs, religious leaders, traditional healers, and senior members of the chief's council. Sometimes I refer to these people as the "indigenous," as distinct from the modern sector, or those who have *always* been leaders, in precolonial times.

For example, here's an excerpt from an actual 2009 call for applications to fill slots for youth leaders in a UNAIDS advisory board. The ad asked:

- Are you actively engaged in the response to HIV and AIDS?
- Are you engaged in the youth movement and believe that UNAIDS is an essential part of the action and solution to HIV and AIDS?
- This role is important to improve communication with key communities such as people living with HIV, women, young people, people who use drugs, sex workers, and men who have sex with men (MSM).

The recruitment thus preselects for people who deem UNAIDS "essential"—that is, who think their own societies can't solve the problem. The ad also discourages young people who are not comfortable with these minorities from applying, and their percentage is greater than in the West, as reflected in the illegality of homosexuality throughout much of Africa. The likely result is a skew in the "civil society" that UNAIDS consults when it wants to know how Africans think. So the feedback is therefore misleading and nonrepresentative.

The third problem for the steering committee is that organizations still have to free themselves from bundling. Most comments during the two-day meeting were about the Big Issues: gender, "achieving universal access" to medical services, empowerment, universal testing, gay rights—all excellent per se, but red herrings with African HIV prevention. Yet overall the participants listened to me at this meeting. I never felt I was there as a room ornament. Two months later, on July 8, 2008, a report from the Geneva meeting was sent to all of us on the steering committee. Unfortunately, it read like any other UNAIDS document: the emphasis was in all the wrong places.

These things take time, I keep telling myself after all these years. Ideology can stand tall after haymakers that would bring a real theory down. You need an enveloping environment, an acid-mist tent, to begin dissolving it.

UN Turnaround in the "Deep South"

In January 2009, as a last deliverable for Harvard, our program co-hosted a conference on multiple and concurrent partners in Gaborone, Botswana. By this time the abbreviation MCP was pretty familiar to people in the global AIDS community. In fact, there had been four MCP conferences in the months before ours, in Washington, D.C., in Europe, and in Africa. At a conference in October 2008, USAID officer Shanti Conly said in her welcoming remarks that she wanted to mention the pioneers in MCP: "Ted Green, Martina Morris, Jim Shelton, Helen Epstein, Daniel Halperin." (I had gotten all but Morris initially interested in looking at the multiple partners issue, and I think Shanti knew that.) That acknowledgment was a nice surprise. Shanti used to be a vocal opponent of the ABC approach (except the C).

At the first tea break, Doug Call from PSI came over to shake my hand and more or less apologize to me for the PSI "struggles we went through" in 2003 over the USAID ABC study. "A lot of us now have egg on our faces," he said. "You should see this conference as a vindication and validation of your arguments about multiple partners." This comment increased my esteem for Doug—not so much because he agreed with me, but because he took a courageous step. It has been hard to admit error in the AIDS World, yet he adapted his thinking to the cognitive dissonance that has been building for years. After the first day was over, Shanti made a beeline for me and wanted to know if I was "pleased" with the way things were going so far, if I was "happy." It seemed important to her that I was pleased, and I said I was.

However, I grew rather apprehensive in the weeks leading up to the conference we would be cohosting in Botswana. I still could not quite believe that people from UNAIDS and the World Bank—as well as those we had invited from USAID and contraceptive companies like PSI—could focus on fidelity, at least without subordinating it to condom promotion. But the conference went very well indeed. Fortunately, some of the pioneers in these issues held leadership roles at the conference: David Wilson of the World Bank (a Zimbabwean with vast experience in Africa), Jim Shelton, Helen Jackson of UNAIDS, Daniel Halperin, several African colleagues, and myself. David and others periodically observed that the number of multiple partnerships had been very clearly associated with greater risk of HIV infection for a long time, and now modeling studies suggested that concurrent partners were especially hazardous. We also recognized that the concept of sexual networks is rather difficult to convey to the public, even in mass media. Again, people think about cause-and-effect as a chain—A leads to B—and not in terms of networks. The philosopher Thomas Hobbes inadvertently expressed this limitation in *Leviathan:* "Science is the knowledge of consequences, and the dependence of one fact on another." Not on several others.

There was the issue of polygamy, which is quite common in the hyperepidemic areas, but also elsewhere in Africa. The evidence remains unclear overall about whether polygamous Africans are at significantly greater risk than monogamous ones. In any case, as conference organizers, we knew we would not try to discourage polygamy. In fact, my colleague from the Ubuntu Institute, Cedza Dlamani, and I made arguments for building our programs upon African culture, rather than condemning, confronting, or circumventing it. Lives come first. We all agreed that, whatever our strategy, it must not look like outsiders preaching to Africans to have fewer sex partners.

We spent nearly two days designing plans for a regional campaign as well as a number of local campaigns to discourage multiple ongoing partnerships. We agreed that condoms don't work, at least in southern and eastern Africa, and that fidelity is the best approach. We agreed that programs must clearly present the condom option as subordinate to behavior change. I am quite sure this was the first time organizations like UNAIDS, the World Bank, and PSI formally stated that condoms are less effective than partner reduction or fidelity. In fact, everyone at the conference was already sold on the evidence. Its purpose was to develop action plans for immediate implementation and to review lessons learned to date from MCP programs. We had no time to waste on people who were oblivious to the evidence of what works in African epidemics.

The national AIDS councils of the two worst-hit countries, Botswana and Swaziland, were well represented at the conference, and by this time both had made partner reduction the top priority in their AIDS plans. Both countries also had fidelity campaigns under way—despite a flabbergasting new UNFPA/PSI campaign in Swaziland called "Sex Is Fun," with the theme: "Condoms—where the fun is at!" The conference concluded that our main message should embody fear appeals, like: "Beware! Sex is dangerous" and "Your risk of death jumps with more than one sex partner."

In March 2009, UNAIDS—now with Michel Sidibé as the executive director—released a report based on the conference. And here, for the first time, the UN made behavior change a higher priority than condom promotion. Condoms were now an if-all-else-fails strategy.[5] However, this was a regional report. I doubt many at Geneva headquarters, or UNAIDS in any other part of the globe, would endorse it. The report appeared around the same time as the uproar about the Pope's comments about condoms (detailed at the outset of this book), which not surprisingly drew harsh rebuttals from UNAIDS—that they are the best weapon we have, and so forth—and sharp questions from that reporter about my hubris in contradicting UNAIDS. A few weeks later, in April 2009, UNAIDS released a *second* report. I worried that, after the big dust-up, it might retreat. But this report restated that fidelity was the highest priority in southern Africa and that condoms should only be a safety net.[6] In fact, this report differed from the first one only in adding our meeting agenda and a list of participants.

Backlash: Death for Gays in Uganda?

In October 2009, Ugandan Member of Parliament David Bahati introduced a bill that called for the death penalty for homosexual rape of children. Uganda has long made homosexuality a crime, as do sixty-nine other nations, and currently its courts can theoretically send anyone convicted of gay sex to jail, although during all my years living and working in Africa, I never heard of it actually happening until very recently. The new bill broadened the definition of offenses, however. Simply touching someone could count, for instance, if the intent was sexual. The bill also had a squeal provision. Everyone— including doctors, teachers, pastors, and AIDS professionals—had to report knowledge of homosexual acts to police within twenty-four hours of learning of them or face three years in jail or a large fine. Even parents had to turn in their gay children.

As I've said before, Uganda has not gone through the Western sexual revolution. As soon as I heard of this bill, I went on record telling interviewers it was completely inhumane and unenforceable. It's also dangerous. In a discussion group for anthropologists, I explained that in the real world it would only "drive homosexuality underground, terrorize gay men and women and their loved ones, and justify witch hunts." The callousness of the bill spawned a global uproar, especially because Western gay activists made it seem like the death penalty could be given for simply being gay. In fact, a Ugandan bill had passed without notice in the 1990s that called for the death penalty for pedophile rape, to protect underage girls. But when it became underage boys, Western groups went into action to lessen the penalties for their abusers. Threats of aid termination have come from Sweden and the United States. President Museveni has said that Uganda must "go slow" on this explosive matter (after Secretary Hillary Clinton reportedly told Museveni the bill had to go, period). At the same time, of course, the blunt pressure from abroad has bred local resistance, a determination to see the bill through no matter what.

A few Westerners have charged that this proposed law is evidence that evangelicals are co-opting Uganda policy. Anthropologists might better view this response as cultural push-back, rather like the millenarianism of a cargo cult or a ghost dance movement, as in: "We Africans must return to God's command [as *they* read it] and all this bad stuff will go away. But if we accept the change being forced upon us, we will become as lost as the whites." As this book goes to press, the outcome of this issue remains unclear. My fear is that activists will use this controversy—already presented as "death penalty for gays"—without mentioning this punishment is only for pedophile, penetrative rape—as an excuse to reject the important, broader lessons from Uganda. One can already see this happening on the AIDS electronic discussion groups. After my public comment about justifying witch hunts, one of my perennial critics posted a peevish comment saying, well, of course it was the ABC model that led to "death for gays." However, this time no one responded. A few years ago, many would have endorsed such a sentiment.

The Missing Link in Consistent Condom Use

Condom programs have failed in Africa for a variety of reasons, including the difficulty of getting people to use them consistently. But what if we don't see lower HIV levels even among consistent users? What then? Real-world data on consistent condom use has been hard to come by. Believe it or not, for a long time few of the major standard surveys, including the Demographic and Health Survey, even asked about it, although it was increasingly clear that people had to use condoms consistently if the devices were to have any chance of reducing HIV across a whole populace. Because of critics like myself and Daniel Halperin, Macro (the organization that conducts the DHS) finally added a question about it in 2005.

Now the DHS is supposed to issue periodic reports analyzing key trends. So we waited for the facts about consistent condom use to appear. After four years we'd heard nothing. What was going on? It was hard to believe that internal researchers at Macro would not have run associations and then posted them on the DHS Web site, as they are supposed to with all data they collect. In fact, the site provides tools that let any user perform cross-tabulations and simple analysis of cross-sectional data, such as condom use during last sex, or age of first sex, by factors like age, education level, and rural/ urban residence.[7] Any member of the public should have been able to match up HIV status with consistent condom use. Yet as I write this, the data are still missing.

My colleagues and I wrote to Macro, asking what they had learned. They were evasive. We suspected they had performed this analysis themselves—it was too important to ignore—and if for some strange reason they hadn't, they would likely have done so once they learned well-known troublemakers were poking into this sensitive area. Macro also knew that because taxpayers fund the DHS and its findings are in the public domain, they had to make the raw data available to us. So we got it. But it wasn't easy to work with. Working with our team, a statistics professor at the University of California at San Francisco needed more than a year to carry out the analysis of four countries.

Despite that difficulty, the approach is easy to describe. We simply compared the prevalence of HIV among people in three groups: those who never used condoms, sometimes did, and always did. And we found *no association* between HIV status and consistent condom use. In some cases consistent users had *higher* HIV prevalence than nonusers and in other cases lower. But overall, those who reported using a condom with every sex act were just as likely to have HIV as those who had never used one at all. How was this result possible?

Note that this kind of study shows correlation, not causation. For instance, consistent condom users may take more risks than nonusers. And cross-sectional studies like the DHS do not tell us when a person became infected. Perhaps some became consistent users after they already had HIV. Also, people may lie about condom habits or overestimate their consistency of use.

Some prospective studies have shown that consistent condom use does reduce risk of infection, by approximately 85 percent—although usually in discordant couples and in near-ideal conditions. Our findings do not necessarily contradict these studies, but the key point is: if condoms were really working in Africa, we would probably be seeing some association in the DHS. As other studies have seen, we also found that inconsistent users had the same or greater HIV prevalence than nonusers. Sporadic use seems to offer no protection and correlates with high infection levels. And sporadic use is the norm in Africa and in countries everywhere.

While Macro has sat on this important data for (by now) five years, Westerners continue to promote condoms to Africans as the best AIDS prevention. Why hadn't Macro brought this information into the light? We don't know, but we believe it is because the findings are radioactive for believers in condoms. Yet if there *had* been a correlation, the fact would have been trumpeted all over the planet, even though an association would not prove a causal connection. The nonproof of causation works both ways. In any case we began trying to make these facts known. We submitted an abstract to present these data at the Global Health Council meetings and to the International AIDS Society (IAS) Conference in Vienna in July 2010. Both gatherings rejected our abstract, without comment. These IAS conferences still reserve all the oral presentations and other major attention for condoms, drugs, and "human rights." As my colleague Norman Hearst has said: "I start to see signs of improvement, of paradigm shift, but then every two years we have the IAS Conference and suddenly we are back in the 1980s: condoms, testing, drugs only."

Epilogue

To overturn orthodoxy is no easier in science than in
philosophy, religion, economics, or any of the other
disciplines through which we try to comprehend the
world and the society in which we live.

RUTH HUBBARD
"Have Only Men Evolved"

AIDS has killed millions the world over unnecessarily, and Africans
and others continue to die from it, although it is easily prevented.
Yet so many beliefs about curbing the disease in Africa have rested
on myth, wishful thinking, willful blindness, stereotypes, fear of
career damage, projection of *us* onto *them*, repetition of distortions,
and money-raising lies. Westerners laughed at witch doctors while
promoting the most lethal falsehoods the continent has ever seen.
Indeed, our errors took on a life of their own, powered by a pro-
sex ideology and strong political views about conservative, religious
values, and Bush policies. Although African AIDS was different, it
suited AIDS industry interests to minimize or deny this difference.

The small but growing number of scientists who saw things as
they are came to expect ad hominem attacks and public questions
about their commitment to the poor, to minorities, to women, even to
babies. Meanwhile, as we saw in Elizabeth Pisani's revelatory *Wisdom*

of Whores, other researchers were clued in but kept manipulating the truth to suit their own purposes, telling themselves it was all for the Greater Good. Deadly mistakes became doctrine and persisted in the face of potent evidence to the contrary. These errors remain with us today. For instance, a book appeared in 2008 with the intriguing title *Scientific Errors and Controversies in the U.S. HIV/AIDS Epidemic: How They Slowed Advances and Were Resolved.*[1] Yet the work perpetuates myths about condoms. It reports that the ABC approach to prevention was cynically known in the public-health community as "anything but condoms," or something unscientific that the religious right had forced on scientists.

Moreover, as our 2010 survey showed, ignorance is now widespread in Uganda, after it had led the world out of darkness a generation earlier. Both men and women believed HIV testing the best way to prevent infection, and condoms the second best. Fidelity came much further down the list, and abstinence was last. The promotion of ideologically driven remedies continues in Uganda. What was the main message Ugandans had seen over the past six months? Some 75 percent answered condoms or testing—and no one responded "zero grazing" or "love faithfully." Yet ABC and fidelity are gaining acceptance, if begrudgingly in some quarters. On the one hand, the ABC language has become so hated in the West, almost certainly because of the Bush connotations, that I use it only because Africans like it and still use it, and we see it in many of their official prevention plans. On the other hand, I recently found myself seated beside a person whose words and actions I criticize throughout this book, yet here he was, seeing the light—or at least a glimmer—and coming over to fidelity. If he was changing his mind, I knew that many others were as well.

I've seen this transition on the larger scale too, and not just with UNAIDS and the multiple and concurrent partners conferences. To its great credit, PSI has endorsed the ABC model on its Web site (although distorted claims remain, such as that female condoms are 98 percent effective). PSI is also leading the way at least in Botswana and Swaziland. In Swaziland, in fact, messages on one of its condom packages ask users to avoid multiple concurrent partners and "Circumcise!" I asked PSI/Botswana, which played a very constructive role in our January 2009 conference, whether these messages also appeared on the PSI condom in Botswana. I heard: "We don't mix a condom message with our campaign to discourage MCP." I was also told that the "Sex Is Fun" campaign in Swaziland ran for only two weeks.

In addition, the World Bank is now funding programs in three of the worst epidemics—Swaziland, Botswana, and Lesotho—to discourage multiple concurrent partners. PEPFAR and USAID increasingly focus on multiple ongoing partners and male circumcision in the four nations of southern Africa. In my meetings with PEPFAR and USAID officials in Swaziland and Botswana, I have found them open to the evidence. Some officials are young and relatively new to their positions, so they don't drag along the baggage of commitment to failed policies. They haven't had to change their minds in front of the world's eye.

Remember those myths about African AIDS I listed at the outset of this book? In 2009, Peter Piot, Mark Dybul, and others published an editorial in *The Lancet* called "AIDS: Lessons Learnt and Myths Dispelled." I opened this with trepidation, only to find that condoms were mentioned just once, and in the order of ABC: "Prevention is, of course, about not only technology, but also behaviour. In many countries on several continents, changes in sexual behaviour (such as waiting longer to become sexually active, having fewer partners, and increased condom use) have been followed by reductions in the number of new HIV infections, providing evidence that efforts to change behaviour can and do work."[2] I was almost speechless.

I cannot say it too often: most of the people I have criticized in this book are friends and colleagues who sincerely believe they are doing the right thing in Africa. I know many of them are good-hearted, intelligent, hard-working, and sometimes amazingly self-sacrificing in their efforts to fight AIDS. They are closer to angels than demons, and we cannot demonize them. In fact, if we look upon these errors as evil or stupid, we commit a dangerous blunder ourselves. Something else occurred here, something grave and insidious, and if it can happen in African AIDS, with so many lives at stake, it can happen anywhere. Because ultimately the problem wasn't the people. It was the way our minds work.

At the core was ideology, with its one-channel perspective, emotional logic, social proof, bundling of unrelated issues (at least in Africa), ethnocentrism, and misaligned incentives. Many of my friends felt the lash of the conformity police, shied away from examining their assumptions, and overlooked the hard evidence and the successes on the ground. This mentality can arise almost without our realizing it and breed disasters, and policymakers badly need to guard against it. We have to cultivate the values—such as courage, vigilance, and awareness of our own uncertainties—that protect us from ourselves. Indeed, uncertainties may remain about AIDS in Africa. Despite all the evidence for networks and male circumcision, the difference in HIV rates between southeastern Africa and the rest of the world is so great that I suspect still other, undiscovered factors are at work. According to one theory, African women have a greater viral load than others in the long period between the high-risk window and final onset. We have to keep our minds open. We can't congratulate ourselves on knowing everything.

The confirmation bias remains a daunting hurdle too, for when people commit to acts with devastating effects on others' lives, they often won't admit error regardless of new evidence. The stakes just seem too great, both in terms of others' opinions and their own sense of self-worth. For instance, in the 1980s therapists used repressed-memory techniques and purported to discover bizarre child abuse rings in daycare centers like McMartin in southern California. The practice was faulty, the rings didn't exist, and many fine people suffered—yet few of these therapists ever acknowledged error. Similarly, when DNA evidence reveals the innocence of prisoners, the district attorneys who convicted them typically fight their release and even afterward concoct far-fetched theories of their guilt. Again, the alternative seems too difficult. It involves admitting that their own mistakes destroyed lives. It seems to imply incompetence.

Yet everyone makes mistakes, and the true incompetence lies in pretending one is the first error-free human in history. Moreover, other people are forgiving of acknowledged errors, even major ones. After the Bay of Pigs blunder, President John Kennedy admitted his sole responsibility—and his popularity rose. After the bloody error of Pickett's Charge at the Battle of Gettysburg, Robert E. Lee said: "All this has been my fault. I asked more of my men than should have been asked of them"—few have questioned Lee's ability before or since. N. Wayne Hale Jr. was launch integration manager at NASA when the space shuttle *Columbia* exploded. "I am guilty of allowing the *Columbia* to crash," he acknowledged, and he now holds a higher position in NASA.

Such admissions are painful, but they imply that the individual is trustworthy and will try not to make the same mistake in the future. That's why many—but not all—people respect them. Some embarrassing proportion of my countrymen are more upset by the whistle-blowing over Abu Ghraib than by the torture that was carried out there. And former Defense Secretary Robert McNamara, an old friend of my father, received hate mail for the memoir he wrote shortly before his death, in which he admitted enormous mistakes in conducting the Vietnam War. Yet his lessons could have helped the United States avoid endless combat in Iraq and Afghanistan. I think most people are much less forgiving of self-justifications, which imply falsehood, weakness of character, and persistence in error. It takes courage to reverse course, as well as wisdom and honesty.

We must take a clear-eyed look at what we are doing. We should stop handing out AIDS funding unless recipients know how to spend it effectively. Money alone isn't the solution; in fact, it makes AIDS World bigger, more resistant to self-examination or change, and more demanding of cash. We have to base AIDS prevention on the best evidence, and overall it shows that the risk of HIV infection declines with male circumcision, fewer sexual partners, and especially avoidance of overlapping partners. The evidence is clearest in the hyperepidemics: we have to promote the low-cost programs that we have stigmatized and that have grown popular in Africa despite us. Momentum is growing for fidelity and delay, but bias against them still pervades implementers on the ground..

We can't shift attention and resources away from those at high risk, including the powerless, oppressed, exploited, raped, and abused. But if we characterize African AIDS victims this way, we miss not just the bull's-eye but the wall. We need to look at the target head-on. Most resources in Africa must go to the majority population, and only some to high-risk groups. If Uganda, with scanty resources in the early years, could design and implement a balanced ABC program, targeting audiences by age, gender, occupation, and other factors, the major donors with billions of dollars can surely do so as well. I have to say one last time: I am staggered by the fact that condoms-testing-drugs has been the formula for all populations in all epidemics, everywhere, even as AIDS advocates see the graveyards fill.

We find the same basic problem with prevention in all three major types of HIV epidemics (heterosexual, homosexual, and injecting drug user): almost all strategies have been risk or harm reduction. We start with the axiom that we cannot—or should not—change sexual and drug-using behaviors, and we then concentrate on reducing the harm from these behaviors. We mop the floor instead of plugging the leak. This helpless attitude breeds death and damage, and it has to change. As I write, the recession seems to have severely cut back funds for PEPFAR, the Global Fund, and indeed most programs except (so far) some charities like the Gates Foundation. We Democrats felt we needed to spend more than Bush, but the thirty-nine billion dollars authorized for AIDS in PEPFAR II was simply authorized, not mandated, and the U.S. government need not actually spend it. Indeed, it seems very unlikely that it will spend an amount even close to thirty-nine billion dollars, and hence some activists have stated publicly that they miss the Bush years. The first casualty is the most expensive category of PEPFAR funding: antiretroviral drugs. New patients needing treatment are finding out that there are no international monies to enroll them, although for the present those patients already enrolled can still get ARVs. Without the drugs they face a slow, wasting death. We will see these haggard sufferers on TV, and as we look at every one of them, we should remember that most Ugandans today think testing and condoms are the best way to stop HIV.

Of course, even without the recession, we should put more resources into prevention than treatment, as we would with any other disease. That's how you save lives. But the current economic slump compels a strategy of fidelity. It's inexpensive, it fits in with African and all culture—even Samoan—and it works. There is simply no alternative. We've spent a quarter century and billions of dollars treating the hyperepidemic with unproven, unsuccessful programs backed by falsehoods and stigmatizing. As a result, countless Africans will soon face AIDS without drugs. We cannot reverse this betrayal.

But we can change our own behavior. It's never too late.

Abbreviations and Acronyms

ABC	Abstain, Be faithful, or use Condoms
ACP	AIDS Control Program
AIDSCAP	AIDS Control and Prevention project
AIDSCOM	AIDS Public Health Communication project
ART	Antiretroviral therapy
ARV	Antiretroviral drug
DHS	Demographic and Health Survey
FBO	Faith-based organization
FGD	Focus group discussion
IDU	Intravenous drug users
JTF	John Templeton Foundation
KAP	Knowledge, attitudes, and practices
MAP	Multi-country HIV/AIDS Program
MC	Male circumcision
MCP	Multiple and concurrent partners
MSM	Men who have sex with men
NIH	National Institutes of Health
NSP	HIV/AIDS National Strategic Plan

OARAC	Office of AIDS Research Advisory Council
OGAC	Office of U.S. Global AIDS Coordinator
PACHA	Presidential Advisory Council on HIV/AIDS
PEPFAR	President's Emergency Plan for AIDS Relief
PSI	Population Services International
RCT	Randomized Controlled Trial
SAGE	Stakeholders Advisory Group, Expanded
SOMARC	Social Marketing for Change
STD	Sexually transmitted disease
STI	Sexually transmitted infection
TRADAP	Traditional Doctors AIDS Project
UAC	Uganda AIDS Commission
UNAIDS	Joint United Nations Programme on HIV/AIDS
UNFPA	United Nations Population Fund
USAID	U.S. Agency for International Development
VCT	Voluntary counseling and testing
WHO	World Health Organization

Notes

Prologue

Epigraph to prologue: Nikki Giovanni, "Of Liberation," in *The Collected Poetry of Nikki Giovanni: 1968–1998* (New York: HarperCollins, 2007), 41.

1. Maureen Dowd, *Bushworld* (New York: Putnam Adult, 2004).

2. Edward C. Green, "The Pope May Be Right," *Washington Post*, March 29, 2009, available online at http://www.washingtonpost.com/wp-dyn/content/article/2009/03/27/AR2009032702825.html.

3. From *BBC Radio Ulster*, Sunday, March 29, 2009.

4. For UNAIDS's admission of statistical errors, see "HIV Data" online at http://www.unaids.org:80/en/KnowledgeCentre/HIVData/default.asp.

5. Edward C. Green, *Rethinking AIDS Prevention: Learning from Successes in Developing Countries* (Westport, Conn.: Praeger, 2003).

6. UNAIDS, "Strategic Considerations for Communications on Multiple and Concurrent Partnerships," March 2009, available online at http://www.unaidsrstesa.org/strategic-considerations-communications-multiple-and-concurrent-partnerships.

7. Edward C. Green and Allison Herling Ruark, *AIDS Behavior and Culture: Understanding Evidence-based Prevention* (Walnut Creek, Calif.: Left Coast Press, 2010).

PART I. THE ROAD TO FIDELITY

Epigraph to Part 1: Jacob Bronowski, *Science and Human Values*, revised ·edition (New York: HarperPerennial, 1990), 61.

Chapter 1. Gangs, Maroons, and the Egg Taboo

1. Susan Sontag, "The Anthropologist as Hero," in *Against Interpretation*, edited by Susan Sontag, 69–81 (London: Vintage, 1994 [1963]).

Chapter 2. The Visitation

1. Lawrence K. Altman, "Concern over AIDS Grows Internationally," *New York Times*, May 24, 1983, available online at http://www.nytimes .com/1983/05/24/science/concern-over-aids-grows-internationally.html ?sec=health.

2. P. Van de Perre, D. Rouvroy, P. Lepage, et al., "Acquired Immunodeficiency Syndrome in Rwanda," *Lancet* no. 2 (1984): 62–65.

3. Nathan Clumeck et al., "Acquired Immunodeficiency Syndrome in African Patients," *New England Journal of Medicine* 310, no. 8 (February 23, 1984): 492–97.

4. Harm Hospers and Cor Blom, "HIV Prevention Activities for Gay Men in the Netherlands 1983–93," in *The Dutch Response to HIV Pragmatism and Consensus*, edited by T. Sandfort (New York: Routledge, 1998). A 2006 meta-analysis of studies of gay men in Asia found that the response rate to "ever had sex with a man, in lifetime" was typically several times higher than the response rate to "anal sex with another man" in a lifetime. Only a minority of these men had ever engaged in the virus-friendly practice. C. Cáceres, K. Konda, M. Pecheny, et al., "Estimating the Number of Men Who Have Sex with Men in Low- and Middle-income Countries," *Sexually Transmitted Infections* 82 (2006) (supplement 3): iii3–iii9.

5. G. J. P. Van Griensven, E. M. M. Devroome, J. Goudsmit, and R. A. Coutinho, "Changes in Sexual Behaviour and the Fall in Incidence of HIV Infection among Homosexual Men.," *BMJ* 298 (1989): 218–21. G. J. P. Van Griensven, R. A. P. Tielman, J. Goudsmit, et al., "Risk Factors

and Prevalence of HIV Antibodies in Homosexual Men in the Netherlands," *American Journal of Epidemiology* 125 (1987): 1048–57.

6. For more discussion on this, see G. Rotello, *Sexual Ecology: AIDS and the Destiny of Gay Men* (New York: Dutton, 1997).

7. Hospers and Blom, "HIV Prevention Activities," 43.

8. E. C. Green, "AIDS in Africa: An Agenda for Behavioral Scientists," in *AIDS in Africa: The Social and Policy Impact*, edited by Norman Miller and Richard Rockwell (New York: Mellen Press and the National Council for International Health, 1988), 175–96.

PART II. UGANDA

Epigraph to Part 2: Yoweri Museveni's 1991 speech at an international AIDS conference, in Y. K. Museveni, *What Is Africa's Problem?* (Minneapolis: University of Minnesota Press, 2000), 252. I debate this availability issue at http://www.stwr.org/health-education-shelter/dialogue-on-aids-prevention.html.

Chapter 3. The Twenty-five-cent Solution

1. E. C. Green, L. Nkya, and A. Outwater, "Narratives of Sex Workers in a Tanzanian Town," *Global AIDSLINK* 63 (August 2000), six install-ments in a series of articles; this is from the first installment.

2. E. C. Green, "Uganda Consultant Trip Report" (USAID/Uganda), World Learning, Inc., Washington, D.C., March 1993.

3. Martha Ainsworth, L. Fransen, and Mead Over, *Confronting AIDS: Evidence from the Developing World* (Brussels: European Commission, 1998).

4. Daniel Low-Beer, "This Is a Routinely Avoidable Disease," *Financial Times*, November 28, 2003.

5. Arthur Allen, "Sex Change," *The New Republic*, May 27, 2002, available online at http://www.tnr.com/article/sex-change.

6. J. Homsy et al., "Evaluating Herbal Medicine for the Management of Herpes Zoster in HIV Infected Patients in Kampala, Uganda," *Journal of Alternative and Complementary Medicine* 5, no. 6 (1999): 553–65.

7. Green, *Rethinking AIDS Prevention*. R. L. Stoneburner and

D. Low-Beer, "Population-level HIV Declines and Behavioral Risk Avoidance in Uganda," *Science* 304 (2004): 714–18.

8. This is discussed in E. C. Green and Kim Witte, "Can Fear Arousal in Public Health Campaigns Contribute to the Decline of HIV Prevalence?" *Journal of Health Communication* 11 (2009): 245–59.

9. Quoted in Elizabeth Pisani, *The Wisdom of Whores: Bureaucracies, Brothels, and the Business of AIDS* (New York: W. W. Norton, 2008).

10. H. J. Rotfeld, "The Textbook Effect: Conventional Wisdom: Myth and Error in Marketing," *Journal of Marketing*, April 2000, 123, also online at http://www.auburn.edu/~rotfehj/TextbookEffect.pdf.

11. Green and Witte, "Fear Arousal, Sexual Behavior Change, and AIDS Prevention."

12. G. Asiimwe-Okiror, A. A. Opio, J. Musinguzi, E. Madraa, G. Tembo, and M. Carael, "Change in Sexual Behavior and Decline in HIV Infection among Young Pregnant Women in Urban Uganda," *AIDS* 11 (1997): 1757–63.

13. John B. Jemmott, Loretta S. Jemmott, and Geoffrey T. Fong, "Efficacy of a Theory-based Abstinence-only Intervention over Twenty-four Months: A Randomized Controlled Trial with Young Adolescents," *Archives of Pediatric Adolescent Medicine* 164, no. 2 (2010): 152–59.

14. Quoted in 2003 article by Tom Carter, *Washington Times*, also available at http://www.usaid.gov/press/releases/2003/uganda030313 .html.

15. Ibid.

16. Author interview with anonymized young mother, in D. Kirby and D. Halperin, "Success in Uganda: An Analysis of Behavior Changes That Led to Declines in HIV Prevalence in the Early 1990s" (Scotts Valley, Calif.: ETR Associates, 2008), 9.

Chapter 4. The Crossroads and the Cul-de-sac

1. This data comes from "Concurrency—How Simultaneous Partnerships Help Spread HIV," available online at http://www.aidsmap.com/ cms1065602.aspx.

2. In one study in Rakai, HIV spread during the initial phase in ten

of twenty-three couples in a cohort; see S. D. Pinkerton, "Probability of HIV Transmission during Acute Infection in Rakai, Uganda," *AIDS and Behavior* 12, no. 5 (2007): 677–84. Another study in Quebec found that half of all transmissions occurred in this period; see Bluma G. Brenner et al., "High Rates of Forward Transmission Events after Acute/Early HIV-1 Infection," *Journal of Infectious Diseases* 195 (2007): 951–59.

3. See Green, *Rethinking AIDS Prevention*, 164. Martina Morris and Mirjam Kretzschmar, "Concurrent Partnerships and the Spread of HIV," *AIDS* 11, no. 5 (April 1997): 641–48.

4. Morris and Kretzschmar, "Concurrent Partnerships and the Spread of HIV."

5. M. Carael, "Sexual Behavior," in *Sexual Behaviour and AIDS in the Developing World*, edited by J. Cleland and B. Ferry (London: Taylor & Francis for the World Health Organization, 1995), 77–123.

6. J. Bongaarts, *Late Marriage and the HIV Epidemic in Sub-Saharan Africa*, Policy Research Division Working Paper no. 216 (New York: Population Council, 2006), 9.

7. E. C. Green, N. Hearst, T. Mah, and A. Herling-Ruark, "Multipartner Sex and the Hyper-Epidemics of Africa," *Studies in Family Planning* 40, no. 1 (2009): 1–8.

8. E. C. Green, B. Zokwe, and J. D. Dupree, *The Role of South African Traditional Healers in HIV/AIDS Prevention and Management* (Arlington, Va.: Family Health International, AIDSCAP Project, 1992).

9. B. Auvert, A. Buvé, E. Lagarde, et al., "Male Circumcision and HIV Infection in Four Cities in Sub-Saharan Africa," *AIDS* 15 (2001): S31–S40. Norman Hearst and Sanny Chen, "Condom Promotion for AIDS Prevention in the Developing World: Is It Working?" *Studies in Family Planning* 35, no. 1 (2004): 39–47.

10. The early scientific studies include R. M. Greenblatt, S. A. Lukehart, F. A. Plummer, T. C. Quinn, C. W. Critchlow, R. L. Ashley, L. J. D'Costa, J. O. Ndinya-Achola, L. Corey, and A. R. Ronald, "Genital Ulceration As a Risk Factor for Human Immunodeficiency Virus Infection," *AIDS* 2, no. 1 (1988): 47–50. J. Bongaarts, P. Reining, P. Way, and

F. Conant, "The Relationship between Male Circumcision and HIV Infection in African Populations," *AIDS* 3, no. 6 (1989): 373–77.

11. E. C. Green, "The Participation of African Traditional Healers in an AIDS/STD Prevention Program," *Tropical Doctor* (1997 suppl. 1): 1–4.

12. E. C. Green, "The Participation of African Traditional Healers in an AIDS/STD Prevention Program," *Tropical Doctor* (1997 suppl. 1): 1–4. E. C. Green, "Male Circumcision and HIV Infection," (letter) *Lancet* 355, no. 9207 (March 11, 2000): 926–27.

13. Gary Slutkin, Sam Okware, Warren Naamara, Don Sutherland, Donna Flanagan, Michel Carael, Erik Blas, Paul Delay, and Daniel Tarantola, "How Uganda Reversed Its HIV Epidemic," *AIDS Behavior* 10, no. 4 (July 2006): 351–60.

14. Douglas Kirby, "Changes in Sexual Behavior Leading to Decline in the Prevalence of HIV in Uganda: Confirmation from Multiple Sources of Evidence," *Sexually Transmitted Infections* 84 (2008): 35–41.

15. J. Shelton and B. Johnston, "Condom Gap in Africa: Evidence from Donor Agencies and Key Informants," *BMJ* 323 (2001), available online at http://www.bmj.com/cgi/content/full/323/7305/139. The data by country were not published in this article, only the summary. The breakdown by country was provided by coauthor Johnston, used with permission here and in 2003 congressional testimony by the author.

16. S. Weller and K. Davis, "Condom effectiveness in reducing heterosexual HIV transmission," *Cochrane Review,* Issue 2, 2004 (Chichester, UK, John Wiley & Sons, Ltd.).

17. S. Ahmed, T. Lutalo, M. Wawer, et al., "HIV Incidence and Sexually Transmitted Disease Prevalence Associated with Condom Use: A Population Study in Rakai, Uganda," *AIDS* 15 (2001): 2,171–79.

18. Saphira Nachizya and Lamba Simpito, "Condoms: The Option in the Fight Against HIV/AIDS," *Times of Zambia,* available online at http://www.times.co.zm/news/viewnews.cgi?category=8&id=1047926671.

19. S. Ahmed et al., "HIV Incidence and Sexually Transmitted Disease Prevalence Associated with Condom Use."

20. A. E. Pettifor, H. V. Rees, A. Steffenson, et al., *HIV and Sexual Behaviour among Youth South Africans: A National Survey of 15–24 Year*

Olds (Johannesburg: Reproductive Health Research Unit, University of Witwatersrand, 2004).

21. Susan Allen et al., "Effect of Serotesting with Counseling on Condom Use and Seroconversion among HIV Discordant Couples in Africa," *BMJ* 304 (June 20, 1992): 1605–9, 1607, available online at http://www.ncbi.nlm.nih.gov/pmc/articles/PMC1881972/pdf/bmj00078-0029.pdf.

22. W. Phoolcharoen, "HIV/AIDS Prevention in Thailand: Success and Challenges," *Science* 280, no. 5371 (1998): 1,873–74.

23. Heng Sopheab, Guy Morineau, Joyce J. Neal, Vonthanak Saphonn, and Knut Fylkesnes, "Sustained High Prevalence of Sexually Transmitted Infections among Female Sex Workers in Cambodia: High Turnover Seriously Challenges the 100 Percent Condom Use Programme," *BMC Infectious Diseases* 8 (2008): 167.

24. As quoted in Apiradee Treerutkuarkul, "Married Women a High-risk Group," *Bangkok Post*, September 9, 2006, available online at http://www.aegis.org/news/bp/2006/BP060903.html.

25. E. C. Green and Aldo Conde, "Sexual Partner Reduction and HIV Infection," (letter) *Sexually Transmitted Infections* 76, no. 2 (2000): 145.

Chapter 5. Infidelity

1. E. C. Green, "Uganda AIDS Study" (letter), *New York Times*, February 26, 2005, A2, available online at http://www.nytimes.com/2005/02/26/opinion/l26aids.html.

2. P. Kajubi, M. R. Kamya, S. Kamya, S. Chen, W. McFarland, and N. Hearst, "Increasing Condom Use without Reducing HIV Risk: Results of a Controlled Community Trial in Uganda," *Journal of Acquired Immune Deficiency Syndromes* 40, no. 1 (2005): 77–82.

3. Vinand Nantulya, quoted in Rod Dreher, "Death in Africa," *National Review*, February 10, 2003, 25–28, 25.

4. Janice A. Hogle, E. C. Green, V. Nantulya, et al. "What Happened in Uganda? Declining HIV Prevalence, Behavior Change, and the National Response," Washington, D.C., U.S. Agency for International Development, 2002, p. 15.

PART III. CALAMITY'S CRADLE

Epigraphs to Part 3: Victor Hugo, *Les Misérables* (New York: Penguin, 1982), 424. William Easterly, *The White Man's Burden: Why the West's Efforts to Aid the Rest Have Done So Much Ill and So Little Good* (New York: Penguin, 2006), 10.

Chapter 6. Putting the Bedroom before the Sickroom

1. Margaret Mead, *Coming of Age in Samoa: A Psychological Study of Primitive Youth for Western Civilisation* (New York: Harper Perennial Modern Classics, 2001). The quotation is from Derek Freeman, *Margaret Mead and Samoa: The Making and Unmaking of an Anthropological Myth* (Cambridge: Harvard University Press, 1986).

2. Derek Freeman, *Margaret Mead and the Heretic: The Making and Unmaking of an Anthropological Myth* (New York: Penguin, 1997).

3. Derek Freeman, *The Fateful Hoaxing of Margaret Mead: A Historical Analysis of Her Samoan Research* (Boulder, Colo.: Westview Press, 1999).

4. Steven Pinker, *How the Mind Works* (New York: W. W. Norton & Company, 1999).

5. Alfred C. Kinsey, Wardell R. Pomeroy, and Clyde E. Martin, *Sexual Behavior in the Human Male* (reprint, Bloomington: Indiana University Press, 1998), 664.

6. Martin Gumpert, "The Kinsey Report," *The Nation*, March 28, 2009, available online at http://www.thenation.com/article/kinsey-report. James H. Jones, *Alfred C. Kinsey: A Public/Private Life* (New York: Norton, 1997).

7. James H. Jones, *Alfred C. Kinsey: A Public/Private Life* (New York: W.W. Norton & Co., 1997).

8. Anne Bolin and Patricia Whelehan, *Perspectives on Human Sexuality* (Albany, N.Y.: SUNY Press, 1999), 32.

9. J. Bancroft, "Alfred C. Kinsey and the Politics of Sex Research," *Annual Review of Sex Research* 15 (2004): 1–39.

10. Theodore Dalrymple, "Tough Love," *City Journal* (Winter 1999), available online at http://www.city-journal.org/html/9_1_oh_to_be.html.

11. Evans as quoted in Andrew Jacobs, "Gays Debate Radical Steps to Curb Unsafe Sex," *New York Times*, February 15, 2005.

12. From http://www.man2manalliance.org/crw/frot/limitnewer.html.

13. Pisani, *Wisdom of Whores*, 308.

14. Theodore Dalrymple, *Romancing the Opiates: Pharmacological Lies and the Addiction Bureaucracy* (New York: Encounter Books, 2008), 102.

15. Randy Shilts, *And the Band Played On* (New York: St. Martin's Press, 1987), 209.

16. Danel Reidpath and Kit Yee Chan, "HIV, Stigma, and Rates of Infection: A Rumor without Evidence," *PLoS Med* 3, no. 10 (2006): e435.

17. "10 Reasons Why Human Rights Should Occupy the Center of the Global AIDS Struggle," Open Society Institute, 2009, available online at http://www.hivhumanrightsnow.org/eng/Reasons/view/9.

18. C. Everett Koop, *The Memoirs of America's Family Doctor* (New York: Random House, 1991), 197–98.

19. Bill Weintraub, "Pansexualism," available online at http://www.heroichomosex.org/crw/defpansexualism.html.

20. Bill Weintraub, personal communication with the author, November 15, 2009.

21. Simon Watney, "The Possibilities of Permutation: Pleasure, Proliferation, and the Politics of Gay Identity in the Age of AIDS," in *Fluid Exchanges: Artists and Critics in the AIDS Crisis*, edited by James Miller (Toronto: University of Toronto Press, 1992), 358.

22. Joshua Lipsman, "Disaster Preparedness: Ending the Exceptionalism," available online at http://www.medscape.com/viewarticle/544741.

23. Ibid.

Chapter 7. Ins and Outs of the Castle

1. From "AIDS Prevention and Paradigms: An Electronic Discussion," online at http://groups.creighton.edu/aarg/prevention.html.

2. Institute of Medicine, *Healthy People 2000: Citizens Chart the Course* (Washington, D.C.: National Academies Press, 1990), 154.

3. From *The Textbook Effect: Conventional Wisdom: Myth and Error in Marketing*, online at http://www.auburn.edu/~rotfehj/TextbookEffect.pdf.

4. Kim Longfield, Megan Klein, and John Berman, "Multi-country

Study on Trusted Partners among Youth: Eritrea, Tanzania, Zambia, and Zimbabwe," Population Services International, Washington, D.C., 2001.

5. The video clip of the Dan Rather interview with Stephen Lewis is available at http://www.hd.net/danrather_epguide.html?page=5.

6. E. C. Green, *Faith-based Organizations: Contributions to HIV Prevention* (Washington, D.C.: USAID/Washington and The Synergy Project, TvT Associates, 2003), available online at http://www.docstoc .com/docs/677395/Faith-Based-Organizations-Contributions-to-HIV -Prevention---USAID-Health-HIVAIDS-Partnerships-Faith-Based -Organizations.

7. Easterly, *White Man's Burden*, 163.

PART IV. SHIFTING THE RIVERBED

Epigraphs to Part 4: Tony Judt, *Ill Fares the Land* (New York: Penguin, 2010), 4–5. Dalrymple, *Romancing the Opiates*, 7. Jean Rostand, *Reflections of a Biologist*, as quoted in James Jaccard and Jacob Jacoby, *Theory Construction and Model-building Skills: A Practical Guide for Social Scientists* (New York: Guilford Press, 2009), 91.

Chapter 8. Jihad

1. Norman Hearst and Sanny Chen, "Condom Promotion for AIDS Prevention in the Developing World: Is It Working?" *Studies in Family Planning* 35, no. 1 (2004): 39–47.

2. Kirby, "Changes in Sexual Behavior Leading to Decline in the Prevalence of HIV in Uganda."

Chapter 9. Breakthrough

1. It was discovered belatedly that neveripine triggers resistance to an important class of anti-HIV drugs, causing problems downstream.

2. Sheryl Gay Stolberg, "The White House Gets Religion on AIDS in Africa," *New York Times*, February 2, 2003. E. C. Green, "The New AIDS Fight: A Plan as Simple as ABC," *New York Times*, March 1, 2003, available online at http://www.nytimes.com/2003/03/01/opinion/ the-new-aids-fight-a-plan-as-simple-as-abc.html, reprinted in slightly shorter form as "Changing Behavior Is Important Too," *International*

Herald Tribune, March 4, 2003, 8, available online at http://www.natap
.org/2003/Retro/day33.htm.

3. Gabriel Rotello, *Sexual Ecology: AIDS and the Destiny of Gay Men*
(New York: Plume, 1997).

4. The Pfizer study was published by Narathius Asingwire et al., "The
District Response Initiative on HIV/AIDS," *Action Research* (August 2003).

5. Presidential Advisory Council on HIV/AIDS (PACHA), *Achieving
an HIV-free Generation: Recommendations for a New American HIV
Strategy* (Washington, D.C.: PACHA, 2005), available online at http://
comminit.com/en/node/220156/347.

6. These studies are discussed in Green, *Rethinking AIDS Prevention.*

7. J. K. B. Matovu, G. Kigozi, and F. Nalugoda, "Repetitive VCT, Sexual Risk Behavior, and HIV-incidence in Rakai, Uganda," presentation
at the Uganda Virus Research Institute, Entebbe, Uganda, November 28,
2003. L. E. Corbett, B. Makamure, Y. B. Cheung, E. Dauya, R. Matambo,
T. Bandason, S. S. Munyati, P. R. Mason, A. E. Butterworth, and R. J.
Hayes, "HIV Incidence during a Cluster-randomized Trial of Two Strategies Providing Voluntary Counselling and Testing at the Workplace,
Zimbabwe," *AIDS* 21 (2007): 483–89. L. Sherr, B. Lopman, M. Kakowa,
et al., "Voluntary Counseling and Testing: Uptake, Impact on Sexual
Behaviour, and HIV Incidence in a Rural Zimbabwean Cohort," *AIDS* 21
(2007): 851–60.

8. J. K. Matovu, V. Ssempijja, F. E. Makumbi, R. H. Gray, G. Kigozi,
F. Nalugoda, D. Serwadda, and M. J. Wawer, "Sexually Transmitted
Infection Management, Safer Sex Promotion and Voluntary HIV
Counselling and Testing in the Male Circumcision Trial, Rakai, Uganda,"
Reproductive Health Matters 15, no. 29 (May 2007): 68–74.

9. A. H. Ruark, E. S. Hudes, J. Goldsmith, E. C. Green, and N. Hearst,
"Knowledge of Positive HIV Status Associated with Increased Consistent
Condom Usage among Married but Not Unmarried Africans," paper
presented at XVIII International AIDS Conference, Vienna, Austria, July
18–23, 2010.

10. A. Creese, K. Floyd, A. Alban, et al., "Cost-effectiveness of HIV/
AIDS Interventions in Africa: A Systematic Review of the Evidence,"
Lancet 360, no. 9336 (2002): 880.

11. See J. D. Shelton, D. T. Halperin, V. Nantulya, et al., "Partner Reduction Is Crucial for Balanced 'ABC' Approach to HIV Prevention," *BMJ* 328 (2004): 891–93. R. L. Stoneburner and D. Low-Beer, "Population-level HIV Declines and Behavioral Risk Avoidance in Uganda," *Science* 304 (2004): 714–18. D. Halperin and H. Epstein, "Concurrent Sexual Partnerships Help to Explain Africa's High HIV Prevalence: Implications for Prevention," *Lancet* 363 (2004): 4–6. Hearst and Chen, "Condom Promotion for AIDS Prevention in the Developing World."

12. D. T. Halperin, M. J. Steiner, M. M. Cassell, et al., "The Time Has Come for Common Ground on Preventing Sexual Transmission of HIV," *Lancet* 364 (2004): 1,913–15.

13. South Africa was best-known then for a youth project called LoveLife program, available online at http://www.lovelife.org.za/.

14. Olive Shisana and Leickness Simbayi, *Nelson Mandela/HSRC Study of HIV/AIDS* (Cape Town: Human Sciences Research Council Publishers, 2002).

15. E. C. Green, *Youth, Empowerment, and Support: The YES! Project, Final Evaluation* (Washington, D.C.: Africare and the Bill and Melinda Gates Foundation, 2004).

16. Green and Ruark, *AIDS, Behavior, and Culture.*

Chapter 10. Policy by Applause

1. Kristin L. Dunkle, Rachel K. Jewkes, Heather C. Brown, Glenda E. Gray, James A. McIntryre, and Siobán D. Harlow, "Gender-based Violence, Relationship Power, and Risk of HIV Infection in Women Attending Antenatal Clinics in South Africa," *Lancet* 363, no. 9419 (May 1, 2004): 1,415–21.

2. Kristin L. Dunkle, Rachel K. Jewkes, Heather C. Brown, Glenda E. Gray, James A. McIntryre, and Siobán D. Harlow, "Transactional Sex among Women in Soweto, South Africa: Prevalence, Risk Factors, and Association with HIV Infection," *Social Science & Medicine* 59, no. 8 (October 2004): 1,581–92.

3. World Health Organization, *Promoting Gender Equality to Prevent Violence against Women* (Geneva: World Health Organization, 2005).

4. Roger England, "Coordinating HIV Control Efforts: What To Do with the National AIDS Commissions," *Lancet* 367 (May 27, 2006): 1,786–89.

5. Nicholas Kristof, "When Marriage Kills," *New York Times*, March 30, 2005, available online at http://www.nytimes.com/2005/03/30/opinion/30kristof.html.

6. The Global Coalition on Women and AIDS, "Preventing HIV Infection in Girls and Young Women," undated, p. 2, available online at http://data.unaids.org/GCWA/gcwa_bg_prevention_en.pdf, italics added.

7. Ministry of Health (Uganda) and ORC Macro, "Uganda HIV/AIDS Sero-Behavioural Survey, 2004–05," Ministry of Health and ORC Macro, Calverton, Md., 2006, p. 106.

8. Stephen Lewis, speech delivered at the Eleventh Conference on Retroviruses and Opportunistic Infections, February 8, 2004, available online at http://www.stephenlewisfoundation.org/news_item.cfm?news=1120.

9. Associated Press, "U.N. Official Blames U.S. for Condom Shortage in Uganda," *USA Today*, August 29, 2005, available online at http://www.usatoday.com/news/world/2005-08-29-us-uganda-aids_x.htm.

10. Lewis as quoted in Mike Pflanz, "Bush 'Damaging the Fight against AIDS,'" *The Telegraph*, August 31, 2005, available online at http://www.telegraph.co.uk/news/worldnews/northamerica/usa/1497314/Bush-damaging-the-fight-against-AIDS.html.

11. These DHS figures come from the Central Bureau of Statistics in Kenya and the Tanzania Commission for AIDS, National Bureau of Statistics and ORC Macro. England, "Coordinating HIV Control Efforts."

12. M. Potts, D. T. Halperin, D. Kirby, A. Swidler, E. Marseille, J. D. Klausner, N. Hearst, R. G. Wamai, J. G. Kahn, and J. Walsh, "Public Health: Reassessing HIV Prevention," *Science* 320, no. 5877 (May 9, 2008): 749–50. N. S. Padian, et al., "Diaphragm and Lubricant Gel for Prevention of HIV Acquisition in Southern African Women: A Randomised Controlled Trial," *Lancet*, online edition (July 13, 2007). R. H. Gray, et al., "Randomised Trials for HIV Prevention," *Lancet*, online edition (July 13, 2007).

13. Raymond S. Nickerson, "Confirmation Bias: A Ubiquitous Phenomenon in Many Guises," *Review of General Psychology* 2, no. 2 (1998): 175–220.

14. The Francis Bacon quote appears in Nickerson, "Confirmation Bias," 176.

15. See http://www.pbs.org/newshour/bb/transportation/july-dec09/othernews_11-25.html.

16. The L. L. Thurstone quote appears in Nickerson, "Confirmation Bias," 176.

Chapter 11. Cracking the Error Edifice

1. Hearst and Chen, "Condom Promotion for AIDS Prevention in the Developing World." Green et al., "Multi-Partner Sex and the Hyper-Epidemics of Africa."

2. Kaye Wellings, Martine Collumbien, Emma Slaymaker, Susheela Singh, Zoë Hodges, Dhaval Patel, and Nathalie Bajos, "Sexual Behaviour in Context: A Global Perspective," *Lancet* 368 (2006): 1,706–28.

3. James Shelton, "Confessions of a Condom Lover," *Lancet* 368, no. 9551 (December 2, 2006): 1,947–49. James Shelton, "Ten Myths and One Truth about Generalised HIV Epidemics," *Lancet* 370, no. 9602 (December 1, 2007): 1,809–11.

4. J. Richens, J. Imrie, and A. Copas, "Condoms and Seat Belts: The Parallels and the Lessons," *Lancet* 355, no. 9201 (2000): 400–403.

5. Michael M. Cassell, Daniel T. Halperin, James D. Shelton, and David Stanton, "Risk Compensation: The Achilles' Heel of Innovations in HIV Prevention?" *BMJ* 332 (2006): 605–7.

6. Green and Witte, "Can Fear Arousal in Public Health Campaigns Contribute to the Decline of HIV Prevalence?" available online at http://www.gwu.edu/~cih/journal/JHClink/v11n3_green.pdf. E. C. Green, D. H. Halperin, Vinand Nantulya, and Janice Hogle, "What Happened to Reduce HIV Prevalence in Uganda?" *AIDS and Behavior* 10, no. 4 (July 2006): 335–46.

7. Craig Timberg, "How AIDS in Africa Was Overstated: Reliance on Data from Urban Prenatal Clinics Skewed Early Projections," *Washington Post*, April 6, 2006, A01. Julie Knoll Rajaratnam, Jake R. Marcus, Alison

Levin-Rector, Andrew N. Chalupka, Haidong Wang, Laura Dwyer, Megan Costa, Alan D. Lopez, and Christopher J. L. Murray, "Worldwide Mortality in Men and Women Aged 15–59 Years from 1970 to 2010: A Systematic Analysis," *Lancet* 375, no. 9727 (May 15, 2010): 1,704–20.

8. UNAIDS, *Evidence for HIV Decline in Zimbabwe: A Comprehensive Review of the Epidemiological Data* (Geneva: UNAIDS, 2005), available online at http://data.unaids.org/publications/irc-pub06/zimbabwe_epi _report_nov05_en.pdf.

9. Mark Dybul as quoted in Erika Check, "HIV Infection in Zimbabwe Falls at Last," *BioEd Online* (February 2, 2006), available online at http://www.bioedonline.org/news/news.cfm?art=2318.

10. T. B. Hallett, J. Aberle-Grasse, G. Bello, et al., "Declines in HIV Prevalence Can Be Associated with Changing Sexual Behavior in Uganda, Urban Kenya, Zimbabwe, and Urban Haiti," *Sexually Transmitted Infections* 82 (2006, suppl. 1): i1–i8.

11. S. Gregson, G. P. Garnett, C. A. Nyamukapa, et al., "HIV Decline Associated with Behavior Change in Eastern Zimbabwe," *Science* 311 (February 3, 2006): 664–66. B. Cheluget, G. Baltazar, P. Orege, M. Ibrahim, L. H. Marum, and J. Stover, "Evidence for Population Level Declines in Adult HIV Prevalence in Kenya," *Sexually Transmitted Infections* 82 (2006 suppl. 1): i21–26. R. Hayes and H. Weiss, "Enhanced: Understanding HIV Epidemic Trends in Africa," *Science* 311, no. 5761 (2006): 620–21. W. Hladik, I. Shabbir, A. Jelaludin, A. Woldu, M. Tsehaynesh, and W. Tadesse, "HIV/AIDS in Ethiopia: Where Is the Epidemic Heading?" *Sexually Transmitted Infections* 82 (2006 suppl. 1): i32–i35.

12. Helen Epstein, *The Invisible Cure: Why We Are Losing the Fight against AIDS in Africa* (New York: Farrar, Straus and Giroux, 2007).

13. Helen Epstein, "The Hidden Cause of AIDS," *New York Review of Books* 49, no. 8 (May 9, 2002).

14. Pisani, *Wisdom of Whores*, 15.

15. Ibid., 271.

16. For the Piot assertion and the Rao quotation, see Ranjit Devraj, "AIDS Scare Reducing Basic Health Funds," *Asia Times,* July 5, 2000, available online at http://www.atimes.com/ind-pak/BG05Df02.html.

17. Seth Mydans, "Low Rate of AIDS Virus in Philippines Is a

Puzzle," *New York Times*, April 20, 2003, available online at http://query
.nytimes.com/gst/fullpage.html?res=9B0CEFDC123AF933A15757C0A
9659C8B63.

18. C. Hermann, E. C. Green, J. Chin, M. Taguiwalo, and C. Cortez,
"Evaluation of the Philippines AIDS Surveillance and Education Project,"
USAID/Philippines, May 8, 2001.

19. Pisani, *Wisdom of Whores*, 11.

20. Ibid., 299.

21. Ibid., 269.

22. "PEPFAR Implementation: Progress and Promise," ix, available
online at http://www.nap.edu/catalog/11905.html.

Chapter 12. Chasing the Wild Programs

1. Rev. Sam Ruteikara, "Let My People Go, AIDS Profiteers,"
Washington Post, June 30, 2008.

2. Ibid.

3. Uganda AIDS Commission, "National HIV and AIDS Strategic
Plan 2007/8-20011/12. Moving towards Universal Access," Kampala,
December 2007, ix.

4. Edward C. Green and Wilfred Mlay, "Let Africans Decide How to
Fight AIDS," *Washington Post*, November 29, 2003, A23, available online
at http://www.washingtonpost.com/ac2/wp-dyn?pagename=article&
node=&contentId=A20298-2003Nov28&notFound=true.

5. For my letter opposing this firing, see E.C. Green, "Do or Dybul:
Was Bush's AIDS Czar a Pragmatic Dissenter, a Tool of the Religious
Right, or Both?" *New Republic*, March 10, 2009, available online at http://
www.tnr.com/politics/story.html?id=ad9380a8-cc6b-423a-8141-6ad34bdd
1772&k-80616.

6. J. Sepulveda, C. Carpenter, J. Curran, et al., "PEPFAR Implementation: Progress and Promise," Institute of Medicine, 2007, available online
at http://www.nap.edu/catalog/11905.html.

7. Ibid., 80.

8. Dan Rather Reports, #312, available online at http://www.hd.net/
transcript.html?air_master_id=A5144.

Chapter 13. A Bridge to Somewhere?

1. Deborah Watson-Jones, Kathy Baisley, Helen A. Weiss, Clare Tanton, John Changalucha, Dean Everett, Tobias Chirwa, David Ross, Tim Clayton, and Richard Hayes, "Risk Factors for HIV Incidence in Women Participating in an HSV Suppressive Treatment Trial in Tanzania," *AIDS* 23 (2009): 415–22. James D. Shelton, Daniel T. Halperin, Vinand Nantulya, Malcolm Potts, Helene D. Gayle, and King K. Holmes, "Partner Reduction Is Crucial for Balanced 'ABC' Approach to HIV Prevention," *BMJ* 328, no. 10 (April 2004): 891–93. Stoneburner and Low-Beer, "Population-level HIV Declines and Behavioral Risk Avoidance in Uganda." Halperin and Epstein, "Concurrent Sexual Partnerships Help to Explain Africa's High HIV Prevalence." Hearst and Chen, "Condom Promotion for AIDS Prevention in the Developing World."

2. See http://www.stwr.org/health-education-shelter/dialogue-on-aids -prevention.html.

3. Paul Farmer, "AIDS and Social Scientists: Critical Reflections," in *Dakar: Senegal*, edited by Charles Becker, Jean-Pierre Dozon, Christine Obbo, and Moriba Touré (Codesria, Karthala & IRD, 1998), 36.

4. Later I would become less certain, however. I'm not sure much has changed at headquarters.

5. UNAIDS, "Strategic Considerations for Communications on Multiple and Concurrent Partnerships."

6. UNAIDS, "Addressing Multiple and Concurrent Partnerships in Southern Africa: Developing Guidance for Bold Action," April 2009, available online at http://www.unaidsrstesa.org/files/u1/MCP_Meeting _Report_Gabarone_28-29_Jan_2009.pdf.

7. See "HIV/AIDS Survey Indicators Database," available online at http://www.measuredhs.com/hivdata/data/start.cfm?survey_type_id =&survey_pop_based=&action=new_table&userid=78414&usertabid =88996&CFID=8254030&CFTOKEN=18304291.

Epilogue

Epigraph to epilogue: Ruth Hubbard, "Have Only Men Evolved," in *The Politics of Women's Biology*, edited by Ruth Hubbard, 87–106 (New

Brunswick, N.J.: Rutgers University Press, 1990). Hubbard is an
emeritus professor of molecular biology at Harvard University.

1. Scott O. Holberg, *Scientific Errors and Controversies in the U.S. HIV/AIDS Epidemic: How They Slowed Advances and Were Resolved* (Westport, Conn.: Praeger, 2008). This book also contains some good points; for instance, it's right about the role of male circumcision.

2. Peter Piot, Michel Kazatchkine, Mark Dybul, and Julian Lob-Levyt, "AIDS: Lessons Learnt and Myths Dispelled," *Lancet* 374, no. 9685 (July 18, 2009): 260–63, 260.

Index

AAAS (American Academy for
  Advancement of Science),
  24–25
Abbot Labs, 116
ABC program
  consensus statement on, 154–156
  IOM report on, 205
  message of, 40–42
  messengers for, 37–40
  overview of in Uganda, 34–40
  policy by applause and, 164
  reasons for success of, 36–37
  USAID and, 141–144, 145–146
  vulnerable groups and, 42–44
ABC vs. CNN Debate, 164
Aborigines gang, 4
abstinence. *See also* Fidelity-
  abstinence programs
  African delegation trip and,
    150–154
  blame game and, 87
  drug addiction programs and,
    102
  fidelity vs., xi–xii, 64
  GAO report on, 206–207

IOM report on, 205–206
myths about, xvi–xvii
omission of from new National
  Strategic Plan (Uganda),
  201–204
PEPFAR and, 147
PEPFAR II and, 207–208
Reproductive Health Matters
  cover and, 187
testimony before House
  subcommittee regarding,
  xiii–xiv, 166
Zambia campaign and, 123–126
abuse. *See* Violence
Academy for Educational Develop-
  ment, 21
Achieving an HIV-Free Generation
  (PACHA), 149
ACP (AIDS Control Program), 37
ActUp, 117
addiction, 101
African AIDS, defined, xi–xii
Africare, 157, 159–160
AIDS, Behavior, and Culture (Green
  and Ruark), xix, 161, 226

AIDS 2031—The Programmatic
Response, 214–218
AIDS Control Program (ACP), 37
AIDS exceptionalism, xviii, 104
AIDS journal, 188
"AIDS: Lessons Learnt and Myths
Dispelled" (Piot et al), 227
AIDS Mafia, 195
*The AIDS Pandemic: The Inter-
section of Epidemiology and
Political Correctness* (Chin), 193
AIDS service organizations
(ASOs), 83, 85
AIDS World
drug companies and, 114–116
faith-based organizations and,
117–120
family planning organizations
and, 114–116
foreign aid and, 127–130
original donors to, 108–111
overview of, x, 107–108
second-level donors to, 111–114
AIDSCAP program, 110–111
AIDSCOM program, 21, 109
AIDSTECH program, 21
Allen, Claude, 145, 156
Altman, Lawrence K., 18
anal sex, 20–21, 85, 99
Anglican Church, 38
annex to National Strategic Plan,
204
"The Anthropologist as Hero"
(Sontag), 6
anthropology, 6–7, 95–97
antiretroviral therapy (ART)
Botswana and, 212
decreased funding for, xix, 231

incidence and, 31
Uganda and, 67, 154
antismoking laws, 89–90
applause, policy by, 163–166
Apuuli, David Kihumuro, 111
ASOs (AIDS service organizations), 83, 85
assault, 167–169
autism, 187

B., Mrs., 123, 125–126
babies, 198
Bacon, Francis, 182
Baer, Hans, 176
Bahati, David, 221–222
Bangkok Global AIDS Confer-
ence, 164–165
Barre-Sinoussi, Francoise, 19
Barton, Tom, 25
bathhouses, 84
behavior change. *See also* Fidelity
AIDSCOM program and, 21
briefing to House Foreign
Affairs Committee on, 206
condom use and, 180
Kenya, Zimbabwe and, 190–192
omission of from new National
Strategic Plan (Uganda),
201–204
PACHA and, 148
Bell, Daniel, 77
Belushi, John, 165
Benedict, Ruth, 79–80
Benedict XVI (Pope), ix–xiii
Bernard, Russ, 11
"Beyond the E^2 = (MC)^3" confer-
ence, 53
bias, 141–142, 181–183

Bill and Melinda Gates Foundation, 137, 159
biology, culture vs., 79–80
birth control, 94, 108. *See also* Condoms
blame game, 87–88, 100, 202–203
blood studies, 200
Boas, Franz, 79–80
Bongaarts, John, 49
Botswana
  bundling and, 93
  condoms and, xv
  fidelity in, 46
  fidelity-abstinence programs and, xix, 211–212, 220
  partner reduction and, 220
  poverty myth and, 177
  Strategic Framework for, 202
Brazil, 164, 186
Break the Chain, 212
bridge grants, 161
bridges to nowhere, 194
Bristol Myers Squibb, 116
Brown, Norman O., 82–83
Buckley, William F., 84
bundling, 90–93, 166, 217–218
Burroughs Wellcome, 117
Burton, Richard F., 174
Bush administration, 145–147

Caldwell, Jack, 138
Call, Doug, 218
CARE International, 108, 166
Careal, Michel, 195
Caritas Internationalis, 119
Castro, Fidel, 36, 136
Cates, Ward, 155
Catholic Church, 118

causation, correlation vs., 168–169, 224
Center for Population Studies (Harvard), 5, 137–138, 142, 161, 214
Chan, Kit Yee, 89–90
Chen, Sanny, 140, 185–186
Chin, Jim, 135, 140, 192–194
China, 197–198
Church of Uganda, 38
circumcision (male), xii, 51–53, 138–139
city dwelling, Rwanda and, 20
civil society, 216–217
clarity, 10
Clinton, Hillary, 204, 222
Clinton, William, 146
Cole, Henry, 133–134
Coming of Age in Samoa (Mead), 78
communities based distribution agents, 69
compassion, 181
compensation, risk and, 51, 187, 188
Conant, Francis, 25
concentrated epidemics, generalized epidemics vs., 215–216
concurrent partnerships, 194, 218–220, 227. *See also* Polygamy
condom officers, 156, 187–188
condoms. *See also* ABC program
  AIDS service organizations and, 85–86
  Botswana and, xv
  defective, 54–56

condoms *(continued)*
  Dominican Republic and, 23–24
  harm reduction and, 100
  Hearst/Chen study and, 140–141
  increasing HIV rates with use
    of, xvii
  lack of consistency in use of,
    55–57
  lack of use of, 58–61
  missing data on consistent use
    of, 222–224
  Pope Benedict XVI controversy
    and, ix–xiv
  randomized control trials and,
    162, 214
  reasons AIDS drop-off in
    Uganda was not caused by,
    53–54
  Reproductive Health Matters
    cover and, 187
  as sex-positive, 98
  social marketing and, 21–24
  statistics on risk reduction by,
    55, 56, 57
  strategy for use of as backfiring,
    33, 35
  Uganda's changing policy on,
    68–69
  unprotected sex myth and,
    178–181
  Yes! Project and, 159
  Zambia campaign and, 122–126
confirmation bias, 181–183, 215,
    228–229
conflicts of interest, 91–92, 115, 117
Conly, Shanti, 218
consensus statement, 154–156
conservatives, defining, 95

consistency, condom usage and,
    54, 55–57
CORE Initiative, 157
corporations, funding and,
    114–117
correlation, causation vs.,
    168–169, 224
corruption, 71, 112
counseling and testing, 150–152,
    154, 179
Crawley William, xii–xiii
critical anthropology, 176–177
cults, 182
cultural relativism, 102–104, 228
culture, biology vs., 79–80

Dalrymple, Theodore, 83
data gap, 72
daycare center example, 229
debut. *See* Sexual debut delay
defects, condom failure and,
    55–56
defilement, 43
delay. *See* Sexual debut delay
despotism of liberty, 98
diaphragms, 179
discordant couples, 55, 57
disease, social forces and, 177
disempowerment of African
    women, myth of, 166–167,
    169–171
disinhibition, 151–152
Dlamani, Cedza, 219
dogma, 173
Dominican Republic, 23–24, 61–62
doomsday cults, 182
Dowse, Tim, 182
Dritz, Selma, 88

drug companies, 116–117, 149
drug use, intravenous, 19, 101
Dugas, Gaetan, 88
Dupont Pharma, 116
Dybul, Mark, 150, 191, 203–204,
    227

$E^2 = (MC)^3$ concept, 51–53
earmarks, 166, 172, 179–180, 204,
    206
Easterly, William, 129–130, 181
economics, 196–198. *See also*
    Funding; Poverty
education, xvii, 33, 43–44, 185
eggs, 12
Eli Lilly, 153
embezzlement, 71, 112
empowerment, 166–167, 169–171
The End of Ideology (Bell), 77
England, Roger, 178
epidemic spread, 193–194
epidemics, generalized vs.
    concentrated, 215–216
Epstein, Helen, 144, 192, 194–195
errors, 186–188, 189–190, 229
ethics, 103
Ethiopia, 165–166, 168
ethnography, 95–97
ethnopornography, 174
Evans, David, 84–85
evidence-based prevention, 113
evidence-informed prevention, 113
exceptionalism, xviii, 104
exponential growth of risk, 48

failure of condoms, 55–56
faith-based organizations (FBOs),
    38, 94, 117–120, 137–138, 146

faithfulness. *See* Fidelity
Family Health International, 108,
    110–111
family planning organizations,
    114–116
famines, 11–12
Farmer, Paul, 161–162, 177, 213
Fauci, Tony, 150, 152
Fay School, 4
FBOs (faith-based organizations),
    38, 94, 117–120, 137–138, 146
Feachem, Richard, 152
fear appeals, 41–42, 109–110, 195
feedback, need for genuine,
    216–217
FHI, 188
fidelity
    abstinence vs., xi–xii, 64
    African delegation trip and,
        150–154
    consensus statement on,
        155–156, 185
    Dominican Republic and,
        61–62
    "Love faithfully" slogan and, 40
    lovers and, 46
    myths about, xvi–xvii, 173–175
    omission of from new National
        Strategic Plan (Uganda),
        201–204
    PEPFAR and, 146–147
    PEPFAR II and, 207–208
    Pope Benedict XVI controversy
        and, xi–xii
    Rwanda and, 189
    sexual freedom vs., 172–173
    studies supporting importance
        of, 192

fidelity *(continued)*
  testimony before House
    subcommittee regarding,
    xiii–xiv, 166
  Uganda's changing policy and,
    69
  women and, 44
fidelity-abstinence programs. *See
  also* ABC program
  in Kenya, xvii–xviii
  PEPFAR II and, 207–208
  Pope Benedict XVI controversy
    and, xiii–xiv
  Swaziland, Botswana and, xix
  in Uganda, xiv, xviii, 31–32,
    66–70
First South African National Youth
  Risk Behavior Survey, 158
fisting, 99
fluids, sexual, 12, 60
foreign aid, 127–130
foreskin, 52
Foucault, Michel, 98
freedom, ideologies of, 98. *See also*
  Sexual freedom
Freeman, Derek, 78–79
Freud, Sigmund, 78
Frist, Bill, 146
funding. *See also* PEPFAR
  drug companies and, 114–116
  Elizabeth Pisani on, 196–198
  faith-based organizations and,
    117–120
  family planning organizations
    and, 114–116
  foreign aid and, 127–130
  implications of fidelity and,
    107–108

Jim Chin on, 193
  lack of correlation with success
    and, 34, 230
  original donors and, 108–111
  PEPFAR II and, 207–208
  second-level donors and,
    111–114
The Futures Group, 21, 108,
    133–134

G., Joe, 16–17, 26
Gallo, Robert, 19
The Gambia, 170
GAO (Government Accounting
  Office) report, 204, 206–207
Gates, Bill, 160, 163–164
Gates Foundation, 137, 159
Gaugin, Paul, 78
Gaultier, Jean-Paul, 195
Gausset, Quentin, 174–175
Gay Men's Health Crisis (GMHC),
    85
gay rights movement, 83–87
Gayle, Helene, 155, 166, 168, 180
gays, 18–21, 80–81, 83–87, 95–96,
    221–222
gender rights, xvii, 90–93, 167–171
generalized epidemics, 215–216
George Washington University, 6
Glaxo-Wellcome, 116
Global AIDS Conferences,
    163–165, 218–221
Global Fund to Fight AIDS,
  Tuberculosis, and Malaria,
    35–36, 71, 112, 207
Good, Charles, 25
Goosby, Eric, 208
Gowan, Ann, 25

Graham, Franklin, 146
Gray, Ron, 151
Greeley, Edward, 15, 25
Green, Adam, 96
Groton, 4
growth rate, 197–198
Gypsies, 120

Haiti, 19, 191
Hale, N. Wayne Jr., 229
Hall, Clarence, 160
Halperin, Daniel
   Harvard project and, 161
   Lancet consensus statement and,
      155
   PEPFAR and, 147
   risk compensation and, 188
   sexual networks and, 219
   USAID and, 138–139
harm elimination, 100–101
harm reduction, 100–102,
   103–104, 230
harm-education strategies, 185
Harper, Charles, 160–161
Harvard, 5, 134–138, 142, 161, 214
hazard pyramid, 49–51
health insurance, 120–121
Health Trust, 125–126
Hearst, Norman, 66–67, 140,
   151–152, 185–186, 201–206
Helms, Jesse, 84, 146
helper T-cells, 19
herpes, 39, 52
heterosexual intercourse, xv–xvi,
   12, 45, 60
high-risk groups, programs for, xv
HIV (human immunodeficiency
   virus), 19

Hobbes, Thomas, 219
Holbrooke, Richard, 150–152
Holland, 20–21
homosexuality, 18–21, 80–81,
   83–87, 95–96, 221–222
hormones, 208–209
House Foreign Affairs Commit-
   tee, 206
House of Representatives,
   testimony before, xiii–xiv, 166
"How Uganda Reversed Its HIV
   Epidemic" study, 53
HTLV-3, 19
Hudes, Esther, 151–152
human immunodeficiency virus
   (HIV), 19
human rights, bundling and,
   90–93
Human Rights Watch, 65–66
Hussein, Saddam, 182
hyperepidemics, xi–xii, 53, 193, 198
hypersexuality, myth of, 173–175

Ibadan University, 137
identity, social, 12
ideology
   bringing to Africa, 104–105
   cultural relativism and, 102–104,
      228
   Elizabeth Pisani on, 196
   harm reduction and, 100–102,
      103–104
   sexual freedom and, 77–78, 83,
      97–100, 103–104
ignorance, outsiders and, 128
immune system, 19
incentives, perverse, outsiders
   and, 129

incidence, overview of, 30–31
income, 20, 33. *See also* Poverty;
　Wealth
India, 197
indicators, 202
Indigenous Theories (Green), 136
Institute of Medicine (IOM), 200,
　204–205
institutionalized prevarication, 79
insurance, 120–121
intercourse, heterosexual, xv–xvi,
　12, 45, 60
International AIDS Society (IAS)
　conferences, 224
International Monetary Fund,
　111–112
International Planned Parenthood
　Association, 61, 164, 178
intravenous drug use, 19, 101
*The Invisible Cure: Why We Are
　Losing the Fight Against AIDS
　in Africa* (Epstein), 194–195
IOM (Institute of Medicine), 200,
　204–205
Iraq policy, 182, 229
Islamic community, 38, 120,
　170–171

Jackson, Helen, 219
Jamaica, 128
jihad, 73–74
Jingxela, Mongezi, 60
John Short and Associates, 21
John Templeton Foundation (JTF),
　160–162
Johns Hopkins University debate,
　135–136, 144
Johnston, Beverly, 53–54

Jong, Erica, 83
journals, 185–188

Kaiser Foundation, 35
KAP (knowledge, attitudes,
　practices) surveys, 138
Kaposi's sarcoma, 18, 19
Kennedy, John F., 229
Kenya, xvii–xviii, 190–192
Kim, James, 177
Kinsey, Alfred, 80–82
Kirby, Doug, 53, 94–95, 135–136,
　143–144, 155
Kissinger, Henry, 3
Kiwanuka, John, 43
Knowledge (journalist), 26
Kolker, Jimmy, 153
Koop, C. Everett, 93–94
Kraft-Ebing, Richard, 78
Kretzschmar, Mirjam, 48
Kristof, Nicholas, 171

Laga, Marie, 195
Laing, R.D., 82–83
The Lancet, 155–156, 186–187, 227
Langerhans cells, 52
LAV (lymphadenopathy-associated
　virus), 18
Lawrence, D.H., 78
Leary, Timothy, 213, 214
Lee, Barbara, xiii–xv, 166, 172,
　179–180
Lee, Robert E., 229
Lesotho, 227
Lewis, Stephen, 91, 115–116, 173,
　208–209
liberals, defining, 95
libertinage, 99

Likoma Island, 46
"Love faithfully" slogan, 40, 67
LoveLife, 157–158
Low-Beer, Daniel, 35–36, 139
Lutaaya, Philly, 39, 41
lymphadenopathy-associated virus
    (LAV), 18

Macro, 223–224
MACRO International, 141
Mah, Timothy, 161
Makerere University, 43, 149
malnutrition, 11–12
Man2Man Alliance, 83–85, 99
Mandela, Nelson, 38
Mandela Study, 158
MAP (Multi-Country HIV/AIDS
    Program), 112
Margaret Mead and the Heretic
    (Freeman), 78–79
Margo, Glen, 109
Marjorie (UNAIDS), 123–126
marketing, 21–24, 31, 63, 115, 133
Maroons, 7–11
marriage, xvii, 115–116, 171–173,
    202–203
Masire, Quett, 211
Matawai people, 7–11, 102–103
mavericks, 195–196
May, Wilfred, 203
McKinnell, Hank, 148–149, 150
McNamara, Robert, 229
MCP. See Multiple and concurrent
    partnerships
Mead, Margaret, 78–80, 174
media, 39, 63–64, 122–126
medications. See Antiretroviral
    therapy

Merck, 116
methadone, 101
microbicides, 179
migratory women, 170
Mogae, Festus, 212
money. See Funding; Poverty
Monico, Sophia Mukasa, 44
Montagnier, Luc, 18–19
morality, 93–94, 102–103
Morris, Martina, 48
Multi-Country HIV/AIDS
    Program (MAP), 112
multiple and concurrent partner-
    ships (MCP), 194, 218–220,
    227. See also Polygamy
Museveni, Yoweri
    Bangkok AIDS conference and,
        164
    homosexuality in Uganda and,
        222
    as leader of Uganda, 30
    on role of condoms, 54, 63–64
    success of Uganda program and,
        36–44
    Vinand Nantulya and, 136
Muslims, 38, 120, 170–171
myths about AIDS in Africa
    commentaries on, 186–187
    disempowerment of women as,
        166–173
    Lancet editorial (2010) and, 227
    overview of, xvi–xvii, 115–116
    poverty as driving force,
        176–178
    promiscuity, 173–175, 186, 195,
        208–209
    unprotected sex as driver,
        178–181

NACO, 197

Namibia, 168

Nantulya, Vinand, 70, 136–137, 139, 142–143, 216–217

"The National Strategic Frameworks for HIV/AIDS Activities in Uganda for 2000/1–2005/6" (Uganda AIDS commission), 68

National Strategic Plans for AIDS, 68, 71, 201–204

negotiation, 164

Nelson Mandela Study, 158

networks, sexual, 45–46, 48–49, 195

Newsweek cover story (2000), 63

Nickerson, Raymond, 181

Nickles, Don, 150

Niger, 11–12

Nigeria, 137–138

Nkya, Lucy, 29, 176, 178, 179

Nobel Prize, 19, 181

OARAC (Office of AIDS Research Advisory Council), 148

Obote, Milton, 30, 36

OGAC (Office of the U.S. Global AIDS Coordinator), 203–204

Okware, Sam, 41, 201–202

"One Man, One Woman" program, xvii–xviii

O'Neill, Joe, 145, 146

Open Society Institute, 93

Oppong, Yaa, 143

outsiders, foreign aid and, 128

Outwater, Anne, 29

Over, Mead, 33

overconfidence, outsiders and, 128

PACHA (Presidential Advisory Council on HIV and AIDS), 148–149, 205

pansexualism, 98–100

Paramaribo, Suriname, 7–11

partner reduction
importance of, 48–49
Johns Hopkins University debate and, 144
Lancet consensus statement and, 155
PEPFAR II and, 207–208
prevention messages and, 170
UNAIDS conference and, 220

partnerships, concurrent, 194, 218–220, 227. *See also* Polygamy

Patient Zero, 88

peer review process, 185–186

PEPFAR (President's Emergency Plan for AIDS Relief), 86, 104, 146–147, 150, 204–208

perceived severity, 109–110

Perry, Jonathan, 88–89, 100

perverse incentives, outsiders and, 129

Peterson, Anne, 145, 150

Pfizer, 148–149

pharmaceutical companies. *See* Drug companies

Philippines, 192, 197

Pinker, Steven, 80

Piot, Peter, 113, 195, 197, 227

Pisani, Elizabeth, 86, 112–113, 146. *See also The Wisdom of Whores*

Planned Parenthood, 61, 164, 178
Planners, 130, 169
Pneumocystis carinii pneumonia, 18
polarization, 93–94, 155
policy by applause, overview of, 163–166
political economy-oriented anthropology, 176–177
polygamy, 16, 50–51, 218–220. *See also* Multiple and concurrent partnerships
Population Action International, xiv
Population Council, 73
Population Services International, 108
Positive Nation, 117
poverty, xvii, 90–93, 176–178
Powell, Colin, 146
Poz, 117
pregnancy, 12, 60
President's Emergency Plan for AIDS Relief. *See* PEPFAR
prevalence, overview of, 31
prevarication, institutionalized, 79
prevention, 137, 145–146
ProFamilia, 61–62
promiscuity
  author and, 4
  harm reduction and, 101
  history of gay rights movement and, 84
  myth of, 173–175, 186, 195, 208–209
  transmission in Rwanda and, 20
prostitutes, 24, 29, 58–60, 176
proven efficacy, 205

PSI, 115, 142, 227
psychographics, 23

queer theory, 95–96

randomized control trials, 162, 214
Rao, Prasada, 197
rape, 43, 221–222
Rather, Dan, 208
Reagan, Ronald, 38
rebellion, 5
Reich, Michael, 137
Reidpath, Daniel, 89–90
Reining, Priscilla, 25
relativism, cultural, 102–104, 228
religious institutions, 38, 94, 117–120, 137–138, 146
representative polygamy, 16
Reproductive Health Matters, 187
Rethinking AIDS Prevention (Green)
  African delegation trip and, 150
  changes in Uganda and, 65
  Elizabeth Pisani and, 195
  findings of Harvard study and, 144
  impact of, xviii
  Jim Chin and, 193
Richens, John, 186–187
risk compensation, 51, 187, 188
risk factors
  age of sexual debut, 49
  differences in between America and Rwanda, 19–20
  hazard pyramid and, 49–51
  male noncircumcision, 51–53
  number of partners, 48–49

risk factors *(continued)*
overview of, 46–47
viral load, 47–48
risk per act of intercourse, 45, 47
risk reduction, 55–56, 179, 230
Roche, 116
Roman Catholic Church, 38, 94
Rotello, Gabriel, 147
Ruark, Allison Herling, xix, 151–152, 161, 226
Rural Waterborne Disease Project, 16
Ruteikara, Sam, 201–203
Rwanda, 20, 189–190
Rwanda Demographic and Health Survey, 189

Saddam Hussein, 182
safer-sex message, 23, 85
SAGE (Stakeholders Advisory Group, Expanded), 123
Sahel, 11–12
Samoa, 78–79, 174
sampling, surveys and, 81–82
San Francisco AIDS Foundation, 85
sangomas (spirit mediums), 16–17
Saramaka people, 8
Satcher, David, 165
Save the Children, 108
scabies, 29
scandals, 71, 112
scare tactics, 41–42, 109–110, 195
Schoepf, Brooke, 25
Schwartlander, Bernard, 195
Scientific Errors and Controversies in the U.S. HIV/AIDS Epidemic: How They Slowed Advances and Were Resolved (Holmberg), 226
scientific evidence, condoms and, xii–xiii
Seabury, Samuel, 5
self-reporting, 57
Senegal, 170, 199
serial monogamy, 46
sero-surveys, 200
Sewer Rats gang, 3–4
"Sex is Fun" campaign, 220, 227
sex workers, 24, 29, 58–60, 176
sex-positive, 98, 105, 109, 158, 187
sexual debut delay
Mandela Study, LoveLife Study and, 158
PEPFAR II and, 207, 208
Rwanda and, 189
sexual networks and, 49
in Uganda, 31, 43
Sexual Ecology (Rotello), 147
sexual freedom
fidelity vs., 172–173
gays and, 83–87
ideology of, 77–78
Kinsey on, 80–82
Mead on, 78–80
as pillar of AIDS ideology, 97–100, 103–104
Samoa and, 78–79
in United States, 82–83
sexual networks, 45–46, 48–49, 195
Sexually Transmitted Infections article, 143–144
Shanti, 85

Shays, Chris, xvi, 173, 178–179
Shelton, Jim, 53–54, 140–141,
    186–187, 188, 219
Shilts, Randy, 87–88
Short and Associates, 21
Sidibé, Michel, 214–218, 220
Singer, Merrill, 176
sizing, condoms and, 55
social control mechanisms,
    121–122
social engineering, 130
social identity, intercourse and, 12
social marketing, 21–24, 115
SOMARC (Social Marketing for
    Change) program, 22–24, 31,
    133
Sontag, Susan, 6
sorcerers, 60
Soweto, xi
special interest groups, 163
spirit mediums (sangomas),
    16–17
stereotyping, 209
stigma, 89–90, 123
Stoneburner, Rand, 35–36, 107,
    139
storage, condoms and, 55
Stover, John, 139
Strategic Framework for Bo-
    tswana, 202
Strategic Plans, 71, 201–204
Sudan, USAID consulting gig
    in, 15
"sugar daddy" phenomenon, 43,
    110
Summers, Larry, 161
Suriname, 7–11

surveys, 34, 80–81
Swaziland, xix, 16–17, 26, 220, 227
syphilis, 52

taboos, eggs and, 12
Takemi Fellowship, 134–137
Tanprasertsuk, Sombat, 60
Tanzania, 29, 56, 168
technical assistance, 128
Templeton Foundation, 160–162
Tess (DFID), 123–126
testing, victim counseling and,
    150–152, 154, 179
textbooks, 130
Thailand, 58, 59–60, 142
Theroux, Paul, 70
Thompson, Tommy, 150
Thurstone, L.L., 182–183
Tobias, Randall, 150, 153–154, 164
top-down approaches, outsiders
    and, 128–129
Tororo district visit, 154
TRADAP (Traditional Doctors
    Aids Project), 52
traditional healers, 12–13, 16–17,
    39, 51–52, 121–122
transactional sex, 167–168, 194.
    See also Prostitutes
transfusions, 19
transmission mechanism, 19
truck drivers, 29
trust, condom use and, 59, 115
Trusted Partner campaign, 115
typhoid fever, 8

UAC (Uganda AIDS Commis-
    sion), 37, 156, 164

Uganda
ABC program in, 33–40
changing message in, 66–70,
226
foreign influence on policies of,
70–71
homosexuality and, 221–222
increase in prevalence in, 65–66
initial work in, 30–32
message in, 40–42
messengers in, 37–40
National Strategic Plans of, 71,
201
presentation on story of, 139,
156–157
reasons condoms could not have
been responsible for drop-off
of AIDS in, 53–54, 59
success of fidelity-abstinence
program in, xiv, 36–37
vulnerable groups and, 42–44
"Uganda ABC Approach," 146,
153
"Uganda: 'Abstinence-Only'
Programs Hijack AIDS
Success Story" (Human Rights
Watch), 65–66
Uganda AIDS Commission, 37,
156, 164
UNAIDS
Botswana conference and,
218–221
Elizabeth Pisani on, 195–200
funding of, 196–200
Hearst/Chen study and, 140–141
overview of, 112–114
scientific evidence and, xii–xiii

United States Agency for International Development. See
USAID
universal access, 207
UNocracy, 196
unprotected sex myth, 178–181
Upjohn, 116
USAID
ABC study of, 141–144
Daniel Halperin and, 138–139
first consulting gig with, 15
funding of, 109
lack of support of, 118–119
letter to regarding fidelity-
abstinence programs, 32
reversal of position on fidelity
and ABC program, 145–146
SOMARC program and,
22–24
utopian social engineering, 130

vaccines, 187
Viagra, 99
Vietnam War, 6
violence, 167–169
viral load, 47, 228
virginity. See Sexual debut delay
Vitillo, Robert, 119
voluntary counseling and testing
(VCT), 150–152, 154, 179
vulnerable groups, Uganda ABC
program and, 42–44

Warren, Michael, 12–13
Washington Post, 190
wealth, infection rates and, 33,
178

weapons of mass destruction, 182
Weintraub, Bill, 99
Weldon, Dave, 150
West Virginia University, 11
Western society, 70–71, 77–78, 104–105
"What Happened in Uganda?" presentation, 139, 156
whistle-blowing, 195
The White Man's Burden (Easterly), 129–130
Wilson, David, 111, 219
Wilson, Page, 133
The Wisdom of Whores: Bureaucracies, Brothels, and the Business of AIDS (Pisani), 195–200, 225–226
Witte, Kim, 42
women
empowerment and, 169–171
infection rates in, 172
innocent wives and, 198
marriage and, 171–173
migratory, 170
myths about disempowerment of, 166–173
Uganda ABC program and, 42–44
violence and, 167–169
Wood, Elizabeth, 99
World Bank, 33–35, 73, 111–112, 227
World Population Society, 133
World Vision, 120

Yes! Project, 158–159
Youth Advisory Group (YAG), 124–125
youth programs, 42–44, 124–125, 157–160

Zaire, 32
Zambezi River, 125–126
Zambia, xviii, 122–126
Zenilman Anomaly, 162
zero grazing, 40, 67, 202–203, 226
Zimbabwe, 190–192
zombies, 17

About the Author

Edward C. Green is former director of the AIDS Prevention Research Project at the Harvard School of Health and the author of six previous books, including *Rethinking AIDS Prevention, AIDS and STDs in Africa,* and *AIDS, Behavior, and Culture.* For more than 30 years, he has worked in the field of applied anthropology and international health, conducting research in Africa, Southeast Asia, and other parts of the world. He has served on boards of directors and advisory boards for many organizations, including the Presidential Advisory Council for HIV/AIDS, the Office of AIDS Research Advisory Council at the National Institutes of Health, the UNAIDS AIDS 2031 Steering Committee, AIDS.org, and the Global Initiative for Traditional Systems of Health, Oxford University.

Other Books from PoliPointPress

The Blue Pages: A Directory of Companies Rated by Their Politics and Practices, 2nd edition

Helps consumers match their buying decisions with their political values by listing the political contributions and business practices of over 1,000 companies. $12.95, PAPERBACK.

Sasha Abramsky, Breadline USA: The Hidden Scandal of American Hunger and How to Fix It

Treats the increasing food insecurity crisis in America not only as a matter of failed policies, but also as an issue of real human suffering. $23.95, CLOTH.

Rose Aguilar, Red Highways: A Liberal's Journey into the Heartland

Challenges red state stereotypes to reveal new strategies for progressives. $15.95, PAPERBACK.

John Amato and David Neiwert, Over the Cliff: How Obama's Election Drove the American Right Insane

A witty look at—and an explanation of—the far-right craziness that overtook the conservative movement after Obama became president. $16.95, PAPERBACK.

Dean Baker, False Profits: Recovering from the Bubble Economy

Recounts the causes of the economic meltdown and offers a progressive program for rebuilding the economy and reforming the financial system and stimulus programs. $15.95, PAPERBACK.

Dean Baker, Plunder and Blunder: The Rise and Fall of the Bubble Economy

Chronicles the growth and collapse of the stock and housing bubbles and explains how policy blunders and greed led to the catastrophic—but completely predictable—market meltdowns. $15.95, PAPERBACK.

Jeff Cohen, *Cable News Confidential: My Misadventures in Corporate Media*
Offers a fast-paced romp through the three major cable news channels—Fox
CNN, and MSNBC—and delivers a serious message about their failure to cover
the most urgent issues of the day. $14.95, PAPERBACK.

Marjorie Cohn, *Cowboy Republic:*
Six Ways the Bush Gang Has Defied the Law
Shows how the executive branch under President Bush systematically defied the
law instead of enforcing it. $14.95, PAPERBACK.

Marjorie Cohn and Kathleen Gilberd, *Rules of Disengagement:*
The Politics and Honor of Military Dissent
Examines what U.S. military men and women have done—and what their families and others can do—to resist illegal wars, as well as military racism, sexual
harassment, and denial of proper medical care. $14.95, PAPERBACK.

Joe Conason, *The Raw Deal: How the Bush Republicans Plan*
to Destroy Social Security and the Legacy of the New Deal
Reveals the well-financed and determined effort to undo the Social Security Act
and other New Deal programs. $11.00, PAPERBACK.

Kevin Danaher, Shannon Biggs, and Jason Mark,
Building the Green Economy: Success Stories from the Grassroots
Shows how community groups, families, and individual citizens have protected
their food and water, cleaned up their neighborhoods, and strengthened their
local economies. $16.00, PAPERBACK.

Kevin Danaher and Alisa Gravitz, *The Green Festival Reader:*
Fresh Ideas from Agents of Change
Collects the best ideas and commentary from some of the most forward green
thinkers of our time. $15.95, PAPERBACK.

Reese Erlich, *Conversations with Terrorists:*
Middle East Leaders on Politics, Violence, and Empire
Offers critical portraits of six Middle Eastern leaders, usually vilified as terrorists,
to probe the U.S. war on terror and its media reception. $14.95, PAPERBACK.

Reese Erlich, *Dateline Havana:*
The Real Story of U.S. Policy and the Future of Cuba
Explores Cuba's strained relationship with the United States, the island nation's
evolving culture and politics, and prospects for U.S. Cuba policy with the depar-
ture of Fidel Castro. $22.95, HARDCOVER.

Reese Erlich, *The Iran Agenda:*
The Real Story of U.S. Policy and the Middle East Crisis
Explores the turbulent recent history between the two countries and how it has
led to a showdown over nuclear technology. $14.95, PAPERBACK.

Todd Farley, *Making the Grades:*
My Misadventures in the Standardized Testing Industry
Exposes the folly of many large-scale educational assessments through an alternately edifying and hilarious first-hand account of life in the testing business. $16.95, PAPERBACK.

John Geluardi, *Cannabiz:*
The Explosive Rise of the Medical Marijuana Industry
Reveals how a counterculture movement created a lucrative medical marijuana industry with a political wing devoted to full legalization. $15.95, PAPERBACK.

Steven Hill, *10 Steps to Repair American Democracy*
Identifies the key problems with American democracy, especially election practices, and proposes ten specific reforms to reinvigorate it. $11.00, PAPERBACK.

Jim Hunt, *They Said What?*
Astonishing Quotes on American Power, Democracy, and Dissent
Covering everything from squashing domestic dissent to stymieing equal representation, these quotes remind progressives exactly what they're up against. $12.95, PAPERBACK.

Michael Huttner and Jason Salzman, *50 Ways You Can Help Obama*
Change America
Describes actions citizens can take to clean up the mess from the last administration, enact Obama's core campaign promises, and move the country forward. $12.95, PAPERBACK.

Helene Jorgensen, *Sick and Tired:*
How America's Health Care System Fails Its Patients
Recounts the author's struggle to receive proper treatment for Lyme disease and examines the inefficiencies and irrationalities that she discovered in America's health care system during that five-year odyssey. $16.95, PAPERBACK.

Markos Kounalakis and Peter Laufer, *Hope Is a Tattered Flag:*
Voices of Reason and Change for the Post-Bush Era
Gathers together the most listened-to politicos and pundits, activists and thinkers, to answer the question: what happens after Bush leaves office? $29.95, HARD-COVER; $16.95 PAPERBACK.

Yvonne Latty, *In Conflict: Iraq War Veterans Speak Out on Duty, Loss,*
and the Fight to Stay Alive
Features the unheard voices, extraordinary experiences, and personal photographs of a broad mix of Iraq War veterans, including Congressman Patrick Murphy, Tammy Duckworth, Kelly Daugherty, and Camilo Mejia. $24.00, HARDCOVER.

Phillip Longman, *Best Care Anywhere:*
Why VA Health Care Is Better Than Yours, **2nd edition**

Shows how the turnaround at the long-maligned VA hospitals provides a blueprint for salvaging America's expensive but troubled health care system. $15.95, PAPERBACK.

Phillip Longman and Ray Boshara, *The Next Progressive Era*

Provides a blueprint for a re-empowered progressive movement and describes its implications for families, work, health, food, and savings. $22.95, HARDCOVER.

Marcia and Thomas Mitchell, *The Spy Who Tried to Stop a War:*
Katharine Gun and the Secret Plot to Sanction the Iraq Invasion

Describes a covert operation to secure UN authorization for the Iraq war and the furor that erupted when a young British spy leaked it. $23.95, HARDCOVER.

Markos Moulitsas, *American Taliban:*
How War, Sex, Sin, and Power Bind Jihadists and the Radical Right

Highlights how American conservatives are indistinguishable from Islamic radicals except in the name of their god. $15.95, PAPERBACK.

Susan Mulcahy, ed., *Why I'm a Democrat*

Explores the values and passions that make a diverse group of Americans proud to be Democrats. $14.95, PAPERBACK.

David Neiwert, *The Eliminationists:*
How Hate Talk Radicalized the American Right

Argues that the conservative movement's alliances with far-right extremists have not only pushed the movement's agenda to the right, but also have become a malignant influence increasingly reflected in political discourse. $16.95, PAPERBACK.

Christine Pelosi, *Campaign Boot Camp: Basic Training for Future Leaders*

Offers a seven-step guide for successful campaigns and causes at all levels of government. $15.95, PAPERBACK.

William Rivers Pitt, *House of Ill Repute:*
Reflections on War, Lies, and America's Ravaged Reputation

Skewers the Bush Administration for its reckless invasions, warrantless wiretaps, lethally incompetent response to Hurricane Katrina, and other scandals and blunders. $16.00, PAPERBACK.

Sarah Posner, *God's Profits:*
Faith, Fraud, and the Republican Crusade for Values Voters

Examines corrupt televangelists' ties to the Republican Party and unprecedented access to the Bush White House. $19.95, HARDCOVER.

Nomi Prins, *Jacked: How "Conservatives" Are Picking Your Pocket—Whether You Voted for Them or Not*

Describes how the "conservative" agenda has affected your wallet, skewed national priorities, and diminished America—but not the American spirit. $12.00, PAPERBACK.

Cliff Schecter, *The Real McCain: Why Conservatives Don't Trust Him—And Why Independents Shouldn't*

Explores the gap between the public persona of John McCain and the reality of this would-be president. $14.95, HARDCOVER.

Norman Solomon, *Made Love, Got War: Close Encounters with America's Warfare State*

Traces five decades of American militarism and the media's all-too-frequent failure to challenge it. $24.95, HARDCOVER.

John Sperling et al., *The Great Divide: Retro vs. Metro America*

Explains how and why our nation is so bitterly divided into what the authors call Retro and Metro America. $19.95, PAPERBACK.

Mark Sumner, *The Evolution of Everything: How Selection Shapes Culture, Commerce, and Nature*

Shows how Darwin's theory of evolution has been misapplied—and why a more nuanced reading of that work helps us understand a wide range of social and economic activity as well as the natural world. $15.95, PAPERBACK.

Daniel Weintraub, *Party of One: Arnold Schwarzenegger and the Rise of the Independent Voter*

Explains how Schwarzenegger found favor with independent voters, whose support has been critical to his success, and suggests that his bipartisan approach represents the future of American politics. $19.95, HARDCOVER.

Curtis White, *The Barbaric Heart: Faith, Money, and the Crisis of Nature*

Argues that the solution to the present environmental crisis may come from an unexpected quarter: the arts, religion, and the realm of the moral imagination. $16.95, PAPERBACK.

Curtis White, *The Spirit of Disobedience: Resisting the Charms of Fake Politics, Mindless Consumption, and the Culture of Total Work*

Debunks the notion that liberalism has no need for spirituality and describes a "middle way" through our red state/blue state political impasse. Includes three powerful interviews with John DeGraaf, James Howard Kunstler, and Michael Ableman. $24.00, HARDCOVER.

For more information, please visit www.p3books.com.

About This Book

This book is printed on Cascade Enviro100 Print paper. It contains 100 percent post-consumer fiber and is certified EcoLogo, Processed Chlorine Free, and FSC Recycled. For each ton used instead of virgin paper, we:

- Save the equivalent of 17 trees
- Reduce air emissions by 2,098 pounds
- Reduce solid waste by 1,081 pounds
- Reduce the water used by 10,196 gallons
- Reduce suspended particles in the water by 6.9 pounds.

This paper is manufactured using biogas energy, reducing natural gas consumption by 2,748 cubic feet per ton of paper produced.

The book's printer, Malloy Incorporated, works with paper mills that are environmentally responsible, that do not source fiber from endangered forests, and that are third-party certified. Malloy prints with soy and vegetable based inks, and over 98 percent of the solid material they discard is recycled. Their water emissions are entirely safe for disposal into their municipal sanitary sewer system, and they work with the Michigan Department of Environmental Quality to ensure that their air emissions meet all environmental standards.

The Michigan Department of Environmental Quality has recognized Malloy as a Great Printer for their compliance with environmental regulations, written environmental policy, pollution prevention efforts, and pledge to share best practices with other printers. Their county Department of Planning and Environment has designated them a Waste Knot Partner for their waste prevention and recycling programs.